Christine Hill qualified as a state registered physiotherapist in 1970 and subsequently underwent a postgraduate training in paediatrics, working with babies and children for 10 years, and ultimately heading up the children's physiotherapy service as co-superintendent at St Mary's Hospital, London. She also trained in obstetrics, initially with the NCT and then with the Association of Chartered Physiotherapists in Obstetrics and Gynaecology (now renamed as the Association of Chartered Physiotherapists in Women's Health), qualifying as a full member in 1981.

She is one of London's leading ante-natal and babycare gurus, much sought after professionally, and has seen over 5,000 mothers-to-be in her own practice. Christine is married with three grown up children.

CHRISTINE HILL'S
pregnancy
guide

The essential handbook for all expectant mothers

CHRISTINE HILL

with the help of Lorin Lakasing, MD MRCOG

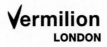

Vermilion
LONDON

7 9 10 8 6

Published in 2009 by Vermilion, an imprint of Ebury Publishing

Ebury Publishing is a Random House Group company

The Random House Group Limited Reg. No. 954009

Addresses for companies within the Random House Group
can be found at www.randomhouse.co.uk

A CIP catalogue record for this book is available from the British Library
Designed and typeset by seagulls.net
Illustrations by Dave Williams @ The Apple Agency Ltd

ISBN 9780091922160

Copies are available at special rates for bulk orders.
Contact the sales development team on 020 7840 8487 for more information.

To buy books by your favourite authors and register for offers, visit
www.randomhouse.co.uk

The information in this book has been compiled by way of general guidance in relation to the
specific subjects addressed, but is not a substitute and not to be relied on for medical, healthcare,
pharmaceutical or other professional advice on specific circumstances and in specific locations.
Please consult your GP before changing, stopping or starting any medical treatment. So far as the
author is aware the information given is correct and up to date as at March 2009. Practice, laws
and regulations all change, and the reader should obtain up to date professional advice on any
such issues. The author and publishers disclaim, as far as the law allows, any liability arising directly
or indirectly from the use, or misuse, of the information contained in this book.

Penguin Random House is committed to a sustainable future for
our business, our readers and our planet. This book is made from
Forest Stewardship Council® certified paper.

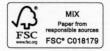

Printed and bound in Great Britain by Clays Ltd, St Ives plc

CONTENTS

ACKNOWLEDGEMENTS

I would like to thank Miss Lorin Lakasing, MD MRCOG, Consultant Obstetrician, St Mary's Hospital, London. Lorin once asked me which pregnancy book I recommended to my patients and that was the start of this. I have been incredibly lucky to have had her help. She has contributed to the chapters (doing rather more than she originally agreed to), answered numerous queries, looked over bits when I had a crisis of confidence and kept me up to date with obstetric practice.

My husband, Professor Peter Hill, FRCP, FRCPCH, FRCPsych, Child and Adolescent Psychiatrist, who, in a professional capacity, helped me get 'bonding' issues factually correct. In a husband's capacity, he supported and helped me with the writing.

I would also like to thank the following for casting an eye over chapters relevant to their expertise:

Barbara Whiteford, MSc, BA, MCSP, SRP, Senior Physiotherapist in Women's Health.

Dr W Aveling, FRCA, Consultant Anaesthetist, University College London Hospital.

Dr Bev Astley, FRCA, Consultant Anaesthetist, University College London Hospital.

John Zinzan, BDS, who for many years has answered my queries regarding dentistry in pregnancy.

Julia Kellaway has been my editor. Yet again, I would like to thank her for her patience and encouragement during the writing of the manuscript.

INTRODUCTION

i'm pregnant for the first time – help!

Unlike other pregnancy books, this book is about you – managing a pregnant life and giving birth – rather than about the miracle of your developing baby.

I hope it will tell you all the things you *really* want to know about the physical and emotional changes that will happen to you during your pregnancy and what giving birth is *really* like. It is also about understanding what happens when you are in labour – including what to do if things don't go to plan and the birth is not straightforward. I am going to try and persuade you to keep an open mind about everything! The book is in a very loose chronological order because women experience various physical problems or face difficult decisions at different times in their pregnancy.

I am a physiotherapist with postgraduate training in paediatrics and obstetrics and have worked all my life with mothers and babies, as well as having had three babies of my own. I have obviously drawn from my professional training. Just as importantly, as an antenatal teacher, I have looked after and listened to the hopes, fears and experiences of over 5,000 pregnant women – many of them medically trained themselves. It has been a privilege to see them through their pregnancies and early motherhood. I have learned so much from them. In many senses, this book has been written by thousands of women, all of whom have had babies themselves.

Pregnancy, childbirth and becoming a parent are remarkable, extraordinary and amazing experiences. And different women, of course, will react and settle into their new pregnancy in different ways, depending upon their personality and circumstances. It may, for instance, be a case of first-time lucky and wonderful news. On the other hand you may have struggled with years of sub-fertility, IVF treatments and miscarriages. You may have felt under pressure from your husband to produce a baby, or this may be a surprise pregnancy with a boyfriend whom you now have to consider as a long-term partner (or not). Everyone's circumstances differ, though there are many common threads.

Whatever your situation, as the news sinks in most of you will feel excitement and the thrill of anticipation. And this is what everyone would expect you to feel. But even those with a perfectly planned pregnancy are likely, at some stage, to experience some unexpected and not entirely comfortable minor misgivings. It is perfectly normal to have any (or all) of the following thoughts:

- How am I going to get through the next months without drinking and partying?
- Have I done the right thing?

- My God – this is a ghastly mistake.
- I'm not ready to have a baby yet.
- Is the baby going to be OK?

During the introductions in my first class, nearly everyone tells me they have one or two of the above worries, even if they have been desperately trying to conceive for ages. For some women these thoughts linger throughout the whole of pregnancy (perhaps with one that comes much later – 'How on earth did I get myself into all this?'). Mixed feelings of excitement and doubt are usual. Yet rather than indicating that you are not yet ready to have a baby, this occasional ambivalence about your pregnancy is quite a good sign. Having a baby is a major life event and adjusting to life events involves a degree of ambivalence. If you have mixed feelings it means that you are intelligently starting to adjust to the major life change ahead and you are beginning to realise that your next year will be very different to any of your previous years. Nearly everything about your present life will change.

Just how you experience your pregnancy will have much to do with what else is going on in your life. I have often taken a new class and looked at a group of beautiful, radiant and self-assured women, about, you might think, to breeze happily through the next few months. But as they start to talk about themselves, a more complicated picture always emerges. It seems that very few women are lucky enough to have a pregnancy precisely the way they planned it, coupled with a trouble-free life devoid of family worries, career crises or money problems!

I don't think I have ever taken a group of women for a first class where more than a third have been in the situation of 'find guy, marry guy, buy/rent home, have baby and live happily ever after'. And if you are not in that fairy-tale category, it's reassuring to know that you are not alone. The most common worries are 'How are we going to manage on only one salary?' or 'How am I going to cope returning to work full-time?'– especially if the baby's father finds he has been made redundant as soon as his partner finds she is pregnant.

What I would like to try and do is provide you with enough information and guidance to help you through those patches when you simply don't know what to do for the best, or have misgivings, micro-panics or serious crises of confidence. I would like to provide support for you – the woman who is now pregnant and extremely anxious to do her absolute best to produce a healthy baby. I will be torn between making some generalisations, whilst also recognising that you and your pregnancy are unique. The aim is to give you enough accurate information to enjoy (or at least make the very best of) your pregnancy, to enjoy whatever sort of birth you may have, but most importantly to enjoy your baby. The finale is not, of course, the birth – and focusing too much on birth is a common mistake. Enjoying your baby is the most important thing of all, but for this to happen you need preparation, confidence and realistic expectations. It can only be a good thing if you can look back on this part of your life as a happy and positive time.

This book will be most useful to those of you who have high expectations and manage a busy life.

I hope I can help you enjoy your pregnancy and your baby while preserving what is special about you as you journey through the next few months, starting with some very practical stuff.

Like so many writers, I have struggled with how best to avoid continually saying 'she or he'. So I call midwives and GPs 'she', and babies, obstetricians and anaesthetists 'he'. This is obviously not always so but it helps to differentiate between them and the mother. I have randomly referred to your birth partner as husband or partner – I realise neither might be the case for some of you.

Consultant Obstetrician Lorin Lakasing has kindly contributed to some of the chapters that follow. To indicate where Lorin is speaking, a different typeface has been used for clarity.

CHAPTER 1

immediate issues

This chapter is about the newly pregnant you, and some of the decisions you may find you have to make. But first, some very practical stuff:

WORKING OUT WHEN YOUR BABY IS DUE

This is a crucial piece of information and worth working out for yourself.

Although it's possible for a pregnancy test to give an early negative result even when you are pregnant, a positive result virtually always (999/1,000) means just that – positively pregnant.

The average length of a pregnancy (gestation) is 38 weeks from conception. So if you now know you are pregnant and if by any chance you know exactly when you conceived, this makes your estimated date of delivery (EDD) pretty easy – count 38 weeks from there.

But life isn't usually this simple – most women don't know exactly when they conceived. Midwives and doctors need to work out how pregnant you are at any time so they can tell how your baby is growing and developing. They use a calculation based on the fact that the majority of women have a 28-day menstrual cycle and will normally ovulate exactly 14 days before their next period is due. So, with a 28-day cycle, ovulation will be both 14 days before her next period and 14 days (two weeks) after the first day of her last period. Conception can only take place around the time of ovulation and there is a window of opportunity of only about three days for this to happen.

Therefore, if you can remember the date of the first day of your last period (and you will be in a minority), the midwife assumes you have a 28-day cycle, ovulated and conceived two weeks after that date, and thus works out when your baby is due by counting 40 weeks (38 plus 2) on. This, incidentally, is why a pregnancy is casually thought of as lasting 40 weeks, rather than the actual 38 weeks.

This method is obviously less accurate if you have a longer or shorter cycle than 28 days. Generally speaking, however long or short your cycle is, women still ovulate 14 days before their next period is due. So if you know your menstrual cycle is 32 days, count 40 weeks from the first day of your last period and add on four days (32 being 4 more days than 28). If your cycle is only 25 days, count 40 weeks from the first day of your last period and take off three days (28 minus 3). It may be about now that it dawns on you that pregnancy undermines your mathematical abilities somewhat.

If you made a note of when your last period started and if your cycle is regular, you can probably just about cope with the above.

But if you didn't (next time round, it's probably worth keeping a note in your diary) or had just come off the pill, which can make the time of ovulation unpredictable, don't worry too much as you are likely to have an ultrasound scan later on at around 11–12 weeks, and this scan will be a pretty accurate way of dating how pregnant you are. Contrary to what you might think, the earlier of the two pregnancy scans (at 11 weeks rather than 20 weeks) is more accurate as far as dating how old your baby is, and therefore when he is due.

And although you probably know this already – the sex of your unborn child is determined by his father.

EARLY WORRIES

Will I Miscarry?

Miscarriages can happen before a woman even knows she is pregnant, so by the time you read this, your risk of miscarriage will be less. It is difficult to be accurate about the number of pregnancies that miscarry, but the figures are pretty high – around 1 in 6, nearly always in the first 12 weeks (first trimester), so you are probably out of the wood on that score. Once you have passed 12 weeks and, more importantly, had a scan which shows a fetal heartbeat, the chance of miscarriage drops considerably. This is why many women prefer not to announce their news to the world until they have hit the 13-week mark.

An early miscarriage (in the first 12 weeks) is therefore not that uncommon. If it happens to you, you will be surprised by the number of girlfriends who tell you they have had the same sad and horrible experience. There is not much you can do to prevent this happening, but to make things more bearable, it might help if you know that the reason for over half of early miscarriages is because something was not right with the fetus. Indeed, if a woman has two miscarriages, the medical assumption is that there was a problem with the fetus rather than the mother. Generally speaking, women are not investigated for any medical causes of miscarriage unless they have had at least two.

Vaginal Bleeding

Bleeding in early pregnancy is common. A very few women will lose a small amount of blood for a couple of days around the time, or just before, their first missed period would otherwise happen. This 'implantation' bleeding occurs as the fertilised egg attaches itself to the lining of the uterus at around 10 days after conception. It does not mean your pregnancy is unstable but can cause confusion as it can be mistaken for a light period. You may wonder whether you are pregnant or not, but a further pregnancy test will tell you.

More commonly, some women (around 20 per cent) experience 'spotting' or occasional light bleeding during the first trimester (especially at the eight-week and twelve-week mark and sometimes after having sex). This can throw you into a panic, but it isn't likely to mean that you are about to have a miscarriage. The vast majority of these women go on to have a perfectly normal pregnancy and baby.

But if you bleed heavily – passing bright red blood or clots – and/or have stomach cramps similar to period pains, you need to contact your GP. Alternatively, most units have 'walk-in' gynae emergency centres.

Ectopic Pregnancy

This is when the fertilised egg implants outside the uterus – and the pregnancy can't progress. It is something that everyone seems to have heard about and therefore worries about but in fact is pretty rare! The symptoms are bleeding and pain, often to one side of your lower tummy area, and it will always be detected by your first scan.

Is My Baby Going to Be OK?

Pretty well all pregnant women worry about this but only a few put it into words. In an antenatal class of fourteen, usually only one woman volunteers that this is on her list of worries. But once she has mentioned it, everyone else nods their head in agreement. It's almost as though it's socially incorrect for a pregnant woman to say she worries about whether her baby is going to be normal. For most women, though, this worry lurks at the back of their mind throughout pregnancy.

It would be stupid to simply reassure you with platitudes, but it might help if you hang on to the fact that 98 per cent of babies are, in fact, perfectly OK. Don't fret that the worry will be a valid premonition; at those rates it can't be. Nor will the act of worrying harm your baby. Some of you may be under stress with an unplanned pregnancy and a faltering relationship, and some of you may have a parent who is ill. If this is the case, you may worry that your unhappy state of mind will harm your baby. Coping with major sadness during your pregnancy is a horrible business, but will not damage your baby or your long-term relationship with him.

As it happens, worrying about your offspring is one of the new things you learn to live with and handle when you become a parent. When your baby is born and is quite normal, you won't give a sigh of relief and say to yourself 'Well that's fine then' and sit back and relax. You will lurch into your baby's first year continuing to worry as to whether he will *remain* OK. And you don't love and worry about your babies any less as they grow up – which is why you may find your own mother slightly irritating. She still loves you and worries about you, and now that you are pregnant she may seem intrusively anxious and just too excited or too interested in your progress. Paradoxically, if you have lost your mother, it is normal to find that you miss her more than ever at this stage in your life. Pregnancy intensifies emotions and all things to do with mothering – even if your own relationship wasn't perfect. You might find your mother is now more often in your dreams. For those of you whose mother has died (however long ago), it is always tough when you are pregnant.

I Didn't Realise I was Going to Feel so Sick and Unwell

Some women sail through the first few months without a hint of nausea while others are feeling sick or throwing up most of the time – not just in the morning. There is no way of telling beforehand which category you are going to fall into. Before you became pregnant yourself you might have secretly thought some of your pregnant girlfriends were making rather a fuss about morning sickness – but nausea is certainly not psychological.

If you are unlucky enough to feel (or be) sick, take heart that many authorities view this as a sign of a stable pregnancy. And however bad it is for you, it is not going to affect your baby. For the vast majority of women the nausea and vomiting will pass at around 14 to 16 weeks. For a very few, it is particularly severe and continues for much longer. This is called hyperemesis and is truly awful – perhaps resulting in hospital admission so you can be rehydrated – but yet again, as long as you get medical help it won't affect your baby.

If you are working, sickness can be especially hard to handle. You probably haven't told anyone that you are pregnant, and you may be faced with trying to get through the day when you are feeling like death and disappearing into the loo every 10 minutes. Unfortunately, there aren't any easy solutions to the problems of trying to work (and managing the journey) when you are feeling like this. The first thing you can do is deal with the practicalities by explaining the problem to your husband and see what he can do to help. Perhaps he could organise the food and prepare whatever you can face for supper. Could he possibly go out of his way to drive you to work and avoid the potential nightmare of you throwing up on the bus? Could you afford a mini-cab for a few weeks (taking a sick-bag with you)?

By all means see if there is anything your GP can suggest but brace yourself for the fact that there is no specified safe remedy that works for everyone. Plenty of people suggest ginger but in my experience most women don't find it terribly helpful. When you have figured out which foods you can actually keep down, carry them round in your handbag with a bottle of water (or whatever else you can drink). The conventional suggestion is dry biscuits, such as water biscuits, but I have been surprised at the range of foods that different women have found to be palatable, so experiment. One girl with hyperemesis arrived at every class with dried nuts and a cold café latte…

Forget about mealtimes, and try and eat small quantities of whatever you can as often as you can. And it would probably be a good idea to cancel any evening social life for the time being, and when you get back from work go to bed or at least lie down somewhere. Hang on in there, and pray that the nausea will pass over the next few weeks, which it does for nearly everyone.

Many women will have absolutely none of the above, but

wonder why I haven't mentioned that it is also common to have a persistent craving for chocolate or something else calorie-laden – this is quite usual as well!

My Breasts are so Sore...

So sore that they are sometimes downright painful and you absolutely don't want them touched – another reason for a conversation with your husband. In fact, this is one of the earliest ways of suspecting pregnancy even before you miss a period – there is a little 'tail' of breast tissue that disappears into your armpit and becomes tender as soon as you conceive. Breast sensitivity tends to disappear after the first trimester.

Some of you will also find, perhaps to your alarm, that you expand a cup size (or more) in the first few weeks of pregnancy, although others will remain exactly the same size. Both situations are normal. If you have to buy a new bra or two now, make sure you get a bigger back size as well as a bigger cup size. Although your breasts won't continue to get much larger during the rest of pregnancy, your ribcage will (see Bras, page 142). At some stage you will also notice that your nipples and the area around them (called the areola) become slightly darker.

And I Need to go to the Loo all the Time

Yes – another irritating problem. During the first few weeks, your uterus enlarges so your bladder, underneath it, can't expand as well as it could when you were not pregnant. This problem is compounded by the fact that your kidneys will produce a little more urine. After 12 weeks, things get better for a while. At around 32 weeks, your (by now heavy) baby will be literally lying on your bladder, so going out can be a bit of a problem. You may find you discover where all the public loos are in your area!

Tired and Emotional?

Even if you are lucky enough not to feel or be sick, in the early weeks most women are surprised to find that rather than feeling 'radiant' they feel pretty lethargic and tired; sometimes so tired that it is difficult to get through the day. If this happens to you, take heart from the fact that things will improve when you hit the 12–14-week mark. It may be difficult for your sensitive husband to realise that this is normal rather than secretly thinking you are a bit of a wimp.

You (and he) might also notice that you develop some personality and emotional changes. It is quite normal to:

- burst into tears for trivial reasons
- find the people you most love quite irritating
- be unable to make decisions
- have difficulty remembering things
- lose some of your old self-confidence
- sleep badly at night
- become more dependent on your husband

And to your surprise – sooner or later you start to find yourself studying baby-gear catalogues.

BE REALISTIC

You may think that you will give up work early on in your pregnancy and at last have some time on your hands. Or you may think that, in any case, when you finally have the baby you will be at home, so you will definitely have time to yourself.

When you have a new baby, it is staggeringly unlikely that you will have time on your hands.

Following on from this, now is really NOT the time to:

- buy a puppy
- sign up for a diploma/degree course
- start up your own business

We Have GOT to Move House

You may be lucky enough or super-organised enough to already live with your partner in a big enough home which is suitable in every way for a new baby. Or you may not! If you are renting and want to move, the situation is reasonably straightforward, but if you already own your flat or house, things can be more complicated. Before you go into panic-mode about the need to move immediately it might be worth bearing in mind the following:

- For the first few months it is only a question of finding space in your bedroom for a Moses basket, crib or pram and storage for some baby gear.
- Your joint earnings may change, affecting what size mortgage you can afford.
- House-hunting is time-consuming, and if both of you are working and one of you is pregnant, finding something suitable is a difficult task.
- Selling and buying a house is not only an expensive business, but takes about as long as a pregnancy and birth.

From what I hear from women who come to antenatal classes, those who are trying to sell, buy or move house during their pregnancy put this very high indeed on their stress list! As everyone knows, the exact timeframe of moving house depends on factors that are not under your control. There is always the possible nightmare of moving house when you are about to deliver – or worse, with a five-day-old baby.

At the very end of pregnancy and directly after giving birth, women like everything at home to be in order and very, very clean. Unless you are living somewhere hopelessly unsuitable, it is probably a better plan to try and sort out a move after your baby has been born.

Should We Get Married?

A few couples may consider this important, or may be under pressure from their parents. But again, before rushing in, bear in mind the following:

- Planning and organising a grand wedding and a party, let alone a possible honeymoon, is a major undertaking.
- You will be in for two major life events within months or weeks of each other – one is enough!

I've seen many women who have decided to have a big wedding before their baby is born and found that their focus has been directed on the wedding rather than the baby. In turn, this means that the process of adjusting to their new baby becomes more rushed, stressful and difficult. From my experience, if you want an immediate marriage, the best option is to have a small civil ceremony – and postpone the party until after your baby has been born.

AND NOW WHAT SHOULD I DO?

At some stage after your period is around two weeks overdue, you will need to book an appointment to see your GP. She should confirm your pregnancy, and is your gateway to your future pregnancy care. Brace yourself, however, for the fact that this just might be a disappointing experience, focusing on administrative issues and a computer screen rather than on you. The good news is you are now eligible for free prescriptions.

You may be given some informative literature, such as 'Emma's Diary' – a pregnancy guide produced by the Royal College of General Practitioners. The contents are of a very high quality, but of necessity written for a broad audience of pregnant women. It is possible that at this stage you might also feel another little wave of disappointment as you realise you have now just joined the ranks of 'pregnant women' and are being sucked onto a conveyor belt. Sometimes the individual concerns of a pregnant woman can be overlooked because everyone's attention is drawn to the miracle of the developing baby inside her, and many women say it crosses their mind at this point that they may be in danger of completely losing their personal identity.

Your GP may ask you where you would like to have your baby (see Where Should I Have My Baby? Making an Informed Choice, page 21) and is the person who will book your first antenatal appointment.

CHAPTER 2

birth issues

As you are settling into your pregnancy, your thoughts will move ahead to the birth itself, and you may find you have some unsettling questions and worries:

- I'm terrified of the birth.
- Where shall I have the baby?
- What sort of birth do I want?
- Should I book into some antenatal classes? Where?

Most of you will have at least two from the list – and another way of looking at it is to transform it into positive **thinking ahead**. This is good news. The alternative to thinking ahead is to block out any thought about the future, bury yourself in your work and forget about the pregnancy and birth, let alone the baby. This frame of mind (denial) is of course one option, but you are likely to run into trouble when your baby is born and have to do too much adjusting in too little time.

It might help to consider various issues in turn.

I'M TERRIFIED OF THE BIRTH

Honestly, honestly, most women are. It's the worry most often mentioned when I see women for their first antenatal class. Even if you start off totally relaxed ('Good heavens, women have been having babies for centuries and my mother and sister had no problems...') one glance at a pregnancy book, let alone the chapter on complications, is probably enough to make you slightly apprehensive.

And there is the occasional girlfriend who feels compelled to tell you about any gruesome or indeed terrifying experience that they, or a friend, or a friend of a friend experienced when they had a baby. *Stay away from these friends for the time being.* Stick to the girlfriends who make you feel good, and tell you how exciting, wonderful and magical their experience of pregnancy, birth and having a baby was. Believe me, this is the truth.

Hang on to the fact that 87 per cent of women are able to have a baby with no problems whatsoever – under a hedge (with a midwife to help!) if necessary. That's a pretty large percentage. The type of labour a woman has is dependent on many factors. A straightforward labour is certainly not dependent on willpower, a high pain threshold or how fit you may be. You are not going to have to take an exam, which you pass or fail, and you are certainly not going to be made to have either a 'natural' childbirth or indeed an epidural if that is not what you want at the time. Some labours are quick and easy, and the women don't need pain relief. The vast majority of women really enjoy their labour (I'm not kidding!).

You will have a midwife with you who has been specially trained to look after you and deliver your baby safely. No-one is into making women suffer when they are in labour, and all hospitals will be able to give you pain relief whenever you might need it.

All that matters about having a baby is that the baby is OK, and that you enjoy it. Therefore it is important to book into some antenatal classes, so you will know what to expect, even if you are medically trained yourself (See Why Go to Antenatal Classes? page 33).

WHERE SHOULD I HAVE MY BABY? MAKING AN INFORMED CHOICE

You may well have already been to see your GP. She may have asked you which local hospital or unit you would like to go to, or if there is no choice, booked you into one. It may be that if she suggested Ambridge General, you happily nodded in agreement. You may already have been given the date for your first hospital appointment there, in which case, fine.

Private obstetric care is a very expensive option so, realistically, most first-time mothers are going to have NHS care. Within the NHS you are supposed to be given as much choice as possible about your pregnancy and birth care so you may find that you have to make a decision as to what sort of unit you would like to book into.

Do you want to have your baby in a hospital in a consultant unit or in a midwife-led unit? And do you want to be looked after during pregnancy by your GP and a midwife, or by just a midwife? Does it matter? These other issues, not to mention what sort of birth experience you are hoping for, may create a whole new set of worries, questions and 'urgent things to do' as you try to take in all the different options and advice.

And once your friends find out that you are pregnant you will discover there is no shortage of advice and warnings from them, some of which are not exactly reassuring. There is a good website called www.birthchoiceuk.com which tells you what is available in your area. To be honest, in many areas there is simply not as much choice as we are led to believe – but this does in some ways make things easier, especially if, like most pregnant women, you find making decisions difficult.

Visiting Hospitals

If you have been given a choice, and you don't know which hospital or unit to go for, it is quite OK to ask to have a look round before you book in. Most hospitals arrange a tour, taking groups of prospective parents round the maternity suite. This is useful, since you will be shown round the delivery rooms (where it is all going to happen) and the postnatal wards. You will get a general feel of the atmosphere, which is terribly important. It might be worth mentioning that, in my experience, women report back that some of the shabbiest hospitals give a first-rate maternity service and vice versa – in other words, seemingly cheerful, kind and patient staff are much more important than a new lick of paint on the walls.

The sort of questions you might want to ask the midwife who shows you round are:

- Is there generally an anaesthetist on site (in case you need an epidural)?
- What sort of paediatric cover can the hospital offer? For example, is there a neonatal or Special Care Baby Unit for very premature babies? (Some hospitals have to transfer premature babies to another hospital.)
- How long do first-time mothers usually stay in hospital after delivery?
- Does the hospital have a Domino scheme (see page 24)?

- How many consultant obstetricians are there in the unit – and are you able to request a consultation with one during your pregnancy if you are worried about something?

You might also want to ask what percentage of the midwives are permanent staff (as opposed to midwives booked through an agency, and who don't necessarily know the hospital). It is also worth checking whether the hospital runs its own antenatal classes.

NHS Care

If you book in to have your baby under the NHS, you will almost certainly see several different midwives for your antenatal check-ups, and during labour you will probably be looked after by yet another midwife.

Generally speaking, you will be offered two options as to where you will have your baby: a consultant unit or a midwife-led unit/birth centre.

Consultant Unit

This is the most usual route for most women, and is otherwise known as the maternity wing of a general hospital. Although you are nominally under the general care of a specific obstetrician and his team, if your labour and delivery are straightforward, you may never come across an obstetrician at all. However, if the midwife has any concerns about you during pregnancy or delivery, or feels that forceps or ventouse (suction) are needed to assist delivery, she will call an obstetrician. If you need an epidural, she will call an anaesthetist.

An hour or so after your baby has been born, you will go to the postnatal ward, which typically has four to six beds, although in some hospitals you can pay for a private or an amenity room (see page 27).

In London, my patients and colleagues tell me the current midwife shortage is noticeable on the postnatal wards, though obviously this varies from hospital to hospital. The usual stay in hospital varies from six to twenty-four hours following a normal delivery and around three to four days (if you are lucky) after a Caesarean section.

Midwife-led Units/Birth Centres (or the Very Occasional GP-led Maternity Unit)

This may be:

- in a hospital near a consultant unit
- in a local hospital where there is no consultant unit
- in its own building

The care here will be from midwives, but not from obstetricians. There will probably be better continuity of antenatal care than in a consultant unit but the care will usually be restricted to relatively straightforward pregnancies and anticipated normal and 'natural' deliveries.

Most midwife-led birth centres go out of their way to try and replicate the feeling of having a home birth by making their units as much like a bedroom (rather than a hospital) as possible. Most of these centres will also have a birthing pool for women who would like to consider a water birth.

Some (but very few) hospitals are able to offer a 'Domino' scheme. This is a fantastic scheme, where a community-based midwife (from a small team) provides both your antenatal and labour care. When you go into labour, one of the team (who you already know and have built up a relationship with) will come to your home, stay with you while you are in labour and take you to hospital when you are ready to give birth and deliver you there. She will come home with you about six hours later.

Is it Worth Going Privately?

There are various options for private maternity care: private obstetric care in an NHS or private hospital; hiring an independent midwife; or booking a private room in an NHS hospital.

Private Obstetric Care in an NHS or Private Hospital

For most women, the cost of having a baby privately (currently around £8,000 in London) means that private obstetric care is simply not an option. It is unusual for women to go privately if they live outside London – there are very few private maternity hospitals, or hospitals and obstetricians who cater for private patients. In London, the midwife shortage is at its most acute and therefore the maternity units are under most strain, which may be why the demand for private care is greater. By paying for private obstetric care, you are able to choose a consultant obstetrician with whom you feel comfortable. Incidentally, an obstetrician is 'elevated' (rather than not being properly qualified) from Dr to Mr, Mrs or Miss when they obtain their MRCOG Membership of the Royal College of Obstetricians and Gynaecologists, which can be confusing!

Your obstetrician will look after you during your pregnancy, and see you for each antenatal appointment. When you go into hospital, although a midwife will look after you during labour, she will let your obstetrician know when you are on the labour ward. Although he won't be holding your hand through the first stage of labour, he may pop in to see you and will be responsible for any decisions that may need to be made. He will be with you towards the end of the first stage of labour and will actually deliver your baby. So you are paying for the privilege of continuity of care, direct access to a senior obstetrician at all times and someone at your delivery who can deal with all eventualities. This, to some women, is the most important factor – being delivered by someone they know and trust.

After your baby has been born, you then have the luxury of your own private room and bathroom. The length of your stay in hospital is longer than with NHS care – usually two days or more following a vaginal delivery and up to five days following a Caesarean section.

Independent Midwives

These are qualified, self-employed midwives working essentially outside the NHS system – though local hospitals occasionally link them into the NHS in various ways. Typically, they support natural childbirth, home birth or water birth approaches and come into their own if you want one of these and find that your local NHS arrangements are unsupportive. They cost roughly between £2,000 and £5,000, to be paid in full by your 36th week. If you have to transfer to hospital care you still pay the full amount.

There are not many independent midwives but they offer a continuity of one-to-one care that is unlikely to be matched by the NHS. The Independent Midwives Association has its own website (www.independentmidwives.org.uk) which enables you to find an independent midwife near you.

As I write, there are still problems with indemnity insurance for independent midwives so you should check with an independent midwife as to whether she is insured.

Doulas

These are private companions who support women during labour and in the first few weeks following birth. They are not qualified to make any medical judgements or to deliver a baby (see Doulas, page 84).

Private Rooms

In some NHS hospitals you can ask to pay for an amenity room for your (probably rather brief) postnatal stay. You might think this would be a good idea if you are going to have a Caesarean section and have to stay for a couple of nights, but actually (in London) you will be on your own in what is effectively a cupboard with no-one to help you lift your baby in and out of his crib. Nearly all women tell me that in this situation a ward is better – at least there will be another mother who can help you.

I Think I'll Have a Home Birth

It is possible your midwife might have suggested this, and you are seized by the idea that it would be really nice to have your baby at home rather than having to go to a hospital. Home births are unusual – only about 2 per cent of all births – and these are mostly second or subsequent babies. Crusaders for home births (and they are certainly around) will argue that it is your right and you can insist. Realistically, your local NHS services may not be well enough staffed with sufficiently experienced midwives to support your home birth, so you may have to engage an independent midwife (see opposite).

The other consideration is safety. The whole area has become irritatingly politicised and it is usual for findings from studies to be presented in a biased way. The bias in advice is nearly always towards home birth, citing a woman's right to choose where and how to have her baby (but oddly, not considering that she might choose to have a Caesarean section).

There are some other considerations:

- You can't have an epidural at home.
- If your baby needs help being born – an assisted delivery – you will probably have to be transferred to hospital, as midwives are not trained to do this.
- It is wise to think about what the transfer time to hospital actually would be if you need it in an emergency – anything over 20 minutes is dubious. (There isn't a flying squad of obstetricians who will dash through your front door at a moment's notice – they disappeared years ago.)

The pluses of having your baby at home are obvious – familiar surroundings, home comforts and an experienced midwife. If this is your second pregnancy and your previous delivery was completely straightforward, things are much more predictable and a home birth might be well worth considering. The oft-repeated statement that home births are as safe as those in hospital applies to these low-risk pregnancies and deliveries. But there still remains a small but serious risk of an unforeseen emergency (see below) needing very urgent medical treatment.

Home birth certainly isn't safe if you have:

- **a serious medical condition**
- **twins**
- **placenta praevia (see page 50)**
- **a breech or transverse presentation (see page 166)**
- **high blood pressure**
- **a previous Caesarean section – for whatever reason**

And if this is your first baby, think very carefully indeed. We know that 87 per cent of women are able to have a perfectly straightforward delivery with the aid of a midwife, but by opting for a home birth for your first baby, you are counting on falling into this percentage. Although women wanting a home birth are carefully screened to confirm that they are 'low risk', this is not a guarantee and there is the unpredictable element. Of course, you can always be transferred from home to hospital, but no woman who is in labour likes to be moved, and several studies have shown that up to 40 per cent of first-time mothers in labour who have opted for a home delivery have needed to transfer to hospital.

No experienced obstetrician I have spoken to has been in favour of a first-time mother opting for a home birth. Very, very occasionally – probably too rarely to show up in group surveys – things go unexpectedly and horribly wrong and you or your baby will need immediate, emergency care that can only be given in hospital.

There are occasional (extremely rare) situations when both you and your baby are at risk, such as a complication when the placenta comes away from the wall of the uterus during birth (severe abruptio placentae). This requires an immediate Caesarean section (within minutes) in order to save both your baby's life and yours. I have taken women for antenatal classes who have had this experience – lying on a trolley with midwives literally running them to theatre. I remember one girl (fit, healthy and normal in every respect) who experienced this. When she was telling me about her labour, she said that all she can remember was her consultant shouting to colleagues, 'This is why I will never agree to a home birth.' Incidentally, both mother and baby were fine, post-operatively.

Obviously, the risks are minuscule, but then so are the risks of catching listeriosis and toxoplasmosis, and you have probably been taking steps to avoid them. There is no evidence that babies born at home are subsequently any different from those born in hospital – your baby will not care whether he is born in your bed, a labour ward or an operating theatre. You are making a choice for yourself, not your baby. A birth centre attached to a hospital or a Domino scheme (see above) seems to me to be a pretty good compromise.

WHAT SORT OF BIRTH DO I WANT?

It really isn't unusual or abnormal to feel nervous about labour and birth, though these anxieties tend to subside as the weeks go by. But for some women, the thought of giving birth is so truly terrifying (tokophobia) that if they become pregnant, their pregnancy is spent literally in terror of birth.

Elective (Planned) Caesareans

It is possible to have an elective (planned) Caesarean section on the NHS, but it is important you know what you are letting yourself in for: a Caesarean section is when the baby is delivered through an incision in the abdominal wall and uterus. It is a surgical operation, which, if planned, normally takes place in a hospital operating theatre.

You might think that opting for an elective Caesarean is a straightforward part of 'a woman's right to choose', which is part of NHS ideology. Yet it was originally assumed that women, given the choice, would choose 'natural' childbirth. The idea that an otherwise fit and healthy woman who is capable of giving birth vaginally might, for her own reasons, choose to have an elective Caesarean is still relatively new and politically incorrect in the eyes of some. Nevertheless, there are an increasing number of women who are choosing to have a Caesarean section rather than go through labour. Just as with the home birth issue, opting for an elective Caesarean for no medical reason has become politicised – possibly coupled with celebrities and the rather irritating 'too posh to push' slogan. Commenting on a survey of obstetricians' wishes for their own births, an obstetrician puts things into perspective by saying, 'A prophylactic Caesarean section [having a C-section to avoid the risks of giving birth] being outrageous has been shattered by the fact that almost a third of female obstetricians would choose it for themselves. These choices should not be discredited simply because they are not the ones that were expected.'

When all goes well, a normal vaginal birth can be an emotionally satisfying and wonderful experience. For some women, childbirth is the most fulfilling thing that they will ever do and they believe that it is an essential part of womanhood. But clearly, this is not true for all women. Perhaps it is important to make it clear that studies also show that you certainly don't have to experience labour pains or natural childbirth in order to fall in love with your baby and have a great long-term relationship with him.

An elective Caesarean is a valid choice for some women though they should make that choice in the knowledge that there is a tiny increase in the risk to themselves and their baby compared with vaginal delivery. Recently, for instance, it has been shown that babies born by Caesarean section before 39 weeks have a slight increase in breathing problems and chest infections. (However, elective Caesareans are usually carried out on straightforward pregnancies at 39 weeks.) The important issue is that if this is the route you would like to go down, you will need to discuss this with an obstetrician.

An elective Caesarean under a general anaesthetic is not a realistic option for the majority of women. All obstetricians prefer to operate under a regional anaesthetic (which means you will be awake) whenever possible, as it is safer for the mother and very much safer for her baby. (When a pregnant woman has a general anaesthetic, her baby is also put to sleep and needs the help of a paediatrician to wake him up when he is born.) A regional anaesthetic involves an injection in the lower spine. This would be an epidural or sometimes a spinal and you don't feel any pain!

Bear in mind that a Caesarean section has some disadvantages over a normal vaginal birth:

- The recovery period is longer than it is following a straightforward vaginal delivery, and your stay in hospital will be longer.
- If this is your second baby, you cannot lift up your older child for a few days.
- You will need to organise help when you come home, as you will not be able to stand for long periods.
- You can't drive for a few weeks afterwards (depending on your car insurance).
- You are more likely to need another Caesarean section for a subsequent birth.

What's a Hypnobirth?

Hypnobirthing (www.hypnobirthing.co.uk) is a technique which uses a form of mild self-hypnosis to calm apprehensions and deal with distractions during labour. You can expect a group course of about five sessions and need a birth partner with you. It cannot guarantee a pain-free birth (of course) and is most suitable for women who have a straightforward labour – so it might be worth considering if this is your second or subsequent pregnancy.

Shall I Have a Water Birth?

Many women find getting into water helpful during labour – and many hospitals and virtually all birthing centres have birthing pools. (Check the hospital you are booked into does have one if this idea appeals to you.) From my experience, how helpful water is to a first-time mother is entirely unpredictable! I have seen many women really determined to use a pool, but when the time came, didn't find the water at all helpful. I remember one woman who even ordered her own pool for the hospital, so determined was she to have a water birth. Later she cheerfully told me, 'As soon as I got in, I knew the only way this would help would be for me to put my head under the water and hold it there.'

Conversely, I have seen many women (seemingly most unlikely candidates for a water birth) who were sure they would have an early epidural. But when it came to the time, they found that their labour was going well, the pool was free, they were persuaded to give it a go and much to their surprise they stayed there until it was time to give birth. 'You're not going to believe this – but I spent all my labour in the pool!'

So, by all means consider this as an option, and keep an open mind. But I can think of no advantages to your baby by actually giving birth to him under the water.

WHY GO TO ANTENATAL CLASSES?

Antenatal classes are *a good thing*, even if you:

- can't face them
- haven't the time
- know enough already

- think ignorance is bliss
- plan to have a Caesarean section

For a start, knowledge is power. The classes are a source of information about pregnancy, birth and babies. Knowing what will happen, what you can do, and what others around you will be doing means it is more likely that you will enjoy your labour and will not be frightened.

Having your first baby is venturing into the unknown and most of your girlfriends who have already had babies will tell you it's better if you know what's in store. Being pregnant and giving birth is a very important time in your life – a time you want to enjoy and remember feeling good about. You certainly don't want to feel frightened or out of control.

Antenatal classes will familiarise you with the basic anatomy and physiology of childbirth – not so you can tell the midwife what to do, but so you are able to understand what is happening. If you know what to expect, you are going to be less apprehensive and more likely to enjoy your labour.

Classes should also teach you how to recognise how labour starts, and when it is important to go to hospital rather than stay at home. Even if you know you will be having a Caesarean, you need to be able to recognise an unexpected start of labour. You learn how to breathe through contractions in order to conserve your energy, the different types of pain relief that are on offer, and how you can make it easier for your midwife to deliver your baby. Honestly, ignorance really isn't bliss when it comes to having a baby. If you are reasonably clued up you will feel less helpless during labour and much better equipped to make decisions.

Going to classes helps to focus your mind on your baby – this has been shown to be important when you bring him home. They are likely to include the basics of what you need to know about looking after a new baby, such as feeding, nappy changing and bathing, which is why they are sometimes called parentcraft classes.

Classes build a social network for you. You will meet other women in the same boat. With any luck, not only will you share your pregnancy and new motherhood with them; you will make life-long friendships. Contact with other new mothers will be both fun and supportive to you during the first few months of your new baby's life (particularly if you are a high-powered career girl who knows she is not going to need them). **Whatever your circumstances, I cannot emphasise enough just how important this will be to you.**

OK, I Need to Book into Classes. Which Ones?

Start by checking out the classes at your hospital or maternity unit – these have the advantage of being taken by the people who are actually going to deliver you, so the information you will get should at least be reasonably relevant! It is also good to be able to familiarise yourself with some professional faces, and there is not usually a fee. There may also be pregnancy yoga or exercise classes in your area, which you could go to in addition to antenatal classes, but these are not a substitute.

The National Childbirth Trust (NCT) is the other obvious avenue to pursue – they run classes virtually everywhere in Great Britain. If you ring the headquarters in London (0300 33 00 770), they will give you details of the booking clerk for your area. Their website address is www.nct.org.uk. The NCT is a charity and trains its own teachers. Most of the teachers will have small children of their own and are from a wide variety of backgrounds, some of them medical. The big advantage of the NCT over hospital classes is that they have really impressive support groups after you have had your baby, which are so important. The classes are subsidised, but there is usually a fee of around £150–£350 depending on where you live and the total hours the courses last. Again, depending on your area, the format of NCT classes varies enormously. Sometimes they are held weekly (usually lasting two hours) over a period of several weeks, either during the day or evening. Some tutors hold all-day sessions over a weekend.

Be very careful you don't sign up to anything where the teacher has a crusade for any particular type of birth or seems to be anti-midwife, anti-doctor or anti-pain relief (and this applies even to some NCT tutors). Nor should your teacher be a breastfeeding fanatic. Occasionally I hear of classes in which even the basics of bottle-feeding 'must not' be mentioned in the classes. We all know that breastfeeding is a good thing, but this fanatical type of mindset is positively dangerous for some babies.

It is important for you that at the end of your course you go into labour with confidence, an open mind and realistic expectations – this means you should be prepared for any type of birth. It doesn't matter in the long run whether you had pain relief or not. An antenatal course should not set you up to feel you have failed in some way if, for example, you end up with a Caesarean section! No classes or special exercises can guarantee a normal, natural or straightforward delivery – the position of the baby determines the labour.

Classes for Couples or for Women Only?

To a certain extent this obviously depends on how involved your partner wants to be. There is, in fact, no evidence to show that men who are heavily involved in their partner's pregnancy and birth make better fathers over the next 30 years as a result of attending antenatal classes. I doubt classes are that powerful.

Having taken classes for both couples and women only, I have found that classes held only for women (but with an additional fathers' evening) are better focused and, above all, much more lively and fun than classes for women with their partners. And it can only be good for your baby if you occasionally double up with laughter. Having men in a class usually inhibits women and the class teacher from discussing any intimate problem in detail (not surprisingly). In any case, let's face it – you, rather than your partner, are the one who is actually going to give birth to your baby. Yes, you will need his help during labour, but his support is more important later, when you come home with your baby.

Most men will want to be with you when you are in labour (but not all – and if he doesn't, it won't mean he will be a useless father). They therefore need to know the anatomy and physiology of childbirth, what they can do to help you during labour, and what they can do to help you afterwards. Men also need to be focused on the impact of pregnancy and a baby and the subsequent change in your relationship. But this can all be explained during a competent fathers' evening. (Most fathers' evenings are held for couples, but directed specifically to the fathers to explain what they can do to help.)

I'm Working – so I Have to Go to Evening Classes

Goodness, this is a statement I've heard so often when girls ring in to ask about classes! And there are very few women who don't work. But however much you love your job, in my experience a full day at work followed by a two-hour (or longer) evening class is not good for either you or your baby.

Before rejecting a daytime class, have a word with your personnel manager. You will probably find that you are legally entitled to take time off for antenatal care – and this includes classes. When your baby is in his twenties, you are unlikely to think 'Thank God I worked until I went into labour.'

One last point – move quickly! All good antenatal courses seem to get horribly booked up. Better to book into a couple early on (at around 14 weeks), do your homework and then cancel one of them later if necessary.

So there are various options when it comes to thinking about where to have your baby. Taking time early in pregnancy to review these options is useful so you can try and decide what's best for you. Your GP or midwife will be giving you regular appointments to monitor your health and your baby's progress. In the following chapter, we look at the type of antenatal tests you can expect to come across.

CHAPTER 3

antenatal care and medical problems
(by Lorin Lakasing)

INVESTIGATIONS

First Trimester

When you first discover you are pregnant, your first port of call should be your GP who will confirm the pregnancy and refer you for antenatal care. In the UK, there are many different types of antenatal care. Most women will have 'shared care' between the GP and the maternity unit in their local hospital. Some women will opt for community-based midwifery care and go on to deliver either in their local birth centre, a hospital-based maternity unit or at home. Some women will choose to be cared for privately by independent midwives, and others will opt for private medical care where they are under the care of a named consultant obstetrician. (For more on different options for antenatal care, see Chapter 2.)

If you have a complicated medical or obstetric history, or if you are particularly risk-averse, the safest and most sensible option is antenatal care and delivery in a hospital maternity unit. Please note that the investigations I am about to discuss below apply to care in the UK only and are based on national guidelines for safe practice. Different countries provide antenatal care in different ways, so I urge you not to be tempted to compare your care with that of your friend who lives in Germany!

Booking Visit

Your first antenatal check-up is usually between eight and twelve weeks' gestation and is usually referred to as the 'booking visit'. During this visit, your midwife or doctor will ask you about your present and past health, and may perform a brief physical examination. Your blood pressure and urine are checked and, in most cases, a 'booking' ultrasound scan of your baby is performed. For most women, this is the first time they 'see' their baby. This scan is done to confirm an ongoing pregnancy, to establish your due date with accuracy (even if you have very regular periods, ultrasound dating is still more accurate), and to check whether you are carrying twins (or more!). You will also have a series of blood and urine tests; what is included in these depends on what type of antenatal care you have opted for. The standard nationally recommended tests are outlined below.

Booking Blood and Urine Tests
- **Full blood count** This test establishes whether you are anaemic or not. Anaemia is a common problem during pregnancy and easily addressed by increasing your iron intake. Almost all

women take multivitamins during pregnancy (only take those specifically designed for pregnant women), and most preparations contain some iron.

- **Blood group** Surprisingly, most people in the UK do not know their blood group. What is of particular importance in pregnancy is the rhesus status. The rhesus negative blood type exists in 15 per cent of Caucasian women, and if the baby's father is Rhesus positive and the baby inherits the father's blood type rather than the mother's, the mother can, in very rare circumstances, develop an immune response against her baby which may have serious consequences. In these cases the mother develops antibodies (small proteins which attach themselves to cells) that attack and damage the fetal red blood cells. This is why rhesus-negative women are offered Anti-D injections at certain points during the pregnancy to prevent them developing this immune reaction against their baby. These injections are usually administered in the third trimester at 28 and 34 weeks' gestation.

- **Antibody screen** This blood test detects the presence of any other antibodies (not just Rhesus) in the mother's bloodstream that might cause her baby harm. These proteins are usually induced by previous pregnancies (especially in the case of Rhesus disease) or previous blood transfusions to the mother. It is also important to know the mother's antibody status because even if she has antibodies that are harmless to the baby, in the event that she requires a blood transfusion, the National Blood Service will need to know about her antibody status so that the best possible match is obtained. Antibody testing occurs at booking, then again in the third trimester, usually between 28 and 34 weeks' gestation.

- **Haemoglobin electrophoresis** This is an analysis of the different types of haemoglobin molecules (the oxygen-carrying part of the red blood cell) and is of particular importance in non-Caucasian women. The two most common conditions that can be identified from this test are sickle-cell anaemia and thalassaemia. These conditions are hereditary so specialist counselling may be offered if a woman is found to have these types of haemoglobin.

- **VDRL/Syphilis serology** Although syphilis is very rare nowadays, it is an infection that is easily treatable, and if untreated there is a small risk of the baby being affected. Therefore it is still a national recommendation that testing for this condition continues.

- **Rubella antibodies** Commonly referred to as 'German measles', this condition is strongly associated with multiple fetal defects, particularly if caught by the mother in the first part of pregnancy. Most women in the UK currently in their childbearing years have been immunised against this condition. However, the relatively recent temporary downturn in the uptake of MMR immunisation shortly after its introduction has resulted in an increased prevalence of rubella in the community. This means that pregnant women who are not immune may have an increased chance of catching rubella from children who have not been immunised themselves.

- **Hepatitis B** Hepatitis B infection (a viral infection of the liver) in the mother is reasonably common and there are multiple protective measures that can be undertaken to prevent transmission of this condition from mother to baby. If a mother is found to be positive for hepatitis, further tests will be carried out to find out how infective she is, and she will be advised accordingly.

- **HIV/AIDS** Although testing for HIV/AIDS was very controversial until recently, most authorities now recognise the value of this screening test. This is because of the enormously beneficial impact that appropriate treatment of the mother has in terms of preventing transmission of the virus across the placenta to the developing baby, and indeed similar transmission through breastfeeding after delivery. Most laboratories offer an 'opt out' policy for HIV screening in pregnancy so you don't absolutely have to have it done.

- **Urine tests** Urine infections are very common in pregnancy and most are easily treated with a short course of antibiotics. If early symptoms are not investigated and treated appropriately, there is a risk of developing pyelonephritis, an infective inflammation of the kidney. This condition may be associated with preterm labour so it is vital that your urine is dip-tested at each antenatal check.

Screening for Down Syndrome

This is a veritable minefield! Even professionals can get confused. Down syndrome is the most common chromosomal abnormality with an overall prevalence of about 1 in 600 pregnancies. The older you are the more likely you are to have an affected baby, so if you are 25 years old you have a 1 in 1,500 chance of having an affected baby, but if you are aged 40, you have a 1 in 100 chance of an affected baby.

In most parts of the UK, hospitals will offer women a screening test for this condition (see below), and usually present the result of this test as either 'low risk' or 'high risk'. If a woman has a 'high risk' result, she is then offered invasive testing such as chorionic villus sampling (where a placental biopsy is taken) or amniocentesis (where some fluid from around the baby is sampled). Laboratory analysis of these samples confirms definitively whether your baby has the condition or not. These specialised invasive tests carry a 1 per cent chance of miscarriage so most women are understandably keen to avoid this. If, unfortunately, the baby is affected, one of the options discussed is termination of pregnancy. About 95 per cent of couples who have the diagnosis of Down syndrome confirmed will opt for termination.

Sounds fairly straightforward so far, but sadly, this is not the case. Different maternity units adopt different methods of screening for the same condition. Some screen on the basis of nuchal translucency alone (a scan test carried out at 11–14 weeks' gestation in which the thickness of skin at the back of the baby's neck is measured). Some maternity units use blood tests alone (a combination of three or four hormone tests from a blood sample taken from you at about 16 weeks' gestation, the 'triple test' or 'quadruple test'). Some use a combination of both nuchal translucency scanning and blood tests (combined testing). This can be done either all together in the first trimester, or split between the scan and one lot of blood tests in the first trimester followed by a second blood test in the second trimester, usually at 16 weeks (interval testing). Each screening method has slightly different detection rates and the high-risk mark can be set to marginally different levels. Which particular test your hospital has chosen to adopt often depends on a host of factors but all hospitals have to examine their own data as to how well the test they have adopted works, and there are clear minimum national standards that should be achieved, irrespective of which tests they use.

I must stress that it is important that you should go with only one method of screening for this condition and stick with it, not comparing your result to your neighbour who might have opted for a very different test even though both tests are screening for the same condition! Otherwise you may end up unnecessarily muddled and worried.

Thankfully, most maternity units have screening co-ordinators whose job it is to advise women about taking these tests, and to help with the subsequent interpretation of the results. With good information and advice, women and their partners rarely make choices they regret, and the key is communicating with the well-informed professionals so you have a realistic impression of what these tests can offer you.

Additional Investigations

There are numerous additional investigations that may be advised in the first trimester depending on your medical or family history. Some common examples are listed below:

- Family history of a hereditary disorder. Some couples have complex genetic histories and may need counselling and special tests.
- Medical disorders you already had before you became pregnant. Some conditions (such as diabetes) need closer monitoring in pregnancy and you may require additional blood tests.
- Medication. Certain drugs you may be taking for longstanding medical disorders may need to be changed over to alternatives that are safer in pregnancy, or have their levels checked as doses in pregnancy may be different.

Second Trimester

During this stage of your pregnancy you will be reviewed on a few occasions, and each time your blood pressure will be measured and your urine dip-tested. In addition, your baby will have the 'anomaly scan'.

Anomaly Scan

Most babies are entirely normal. Sadly, some have structural defects which may be quite minor, such as extra digits, whilst others have more major defects, such as spina bifida. The anomaly scan is performed at 18–23 weeks' gestation in most maternity units because this is the stage of pregnancy at which most major and some minor abnormalities can best be detected. The procedure usually takes 20–40 minutes. If the sonographer is concerned about any of the findings, he or she will refer you to a Fetal Medicine unit where you will be re-scanned by a specialist in Fetal Medicine and advised appropriately.

Additional Investigations

There are comparatively few additional investigations that may be required during the second trimester, and these are usually in women who have previously had complicated pregnancies. For example:

- High blood pressure prior to conception or in a previous pregnancy: specialist scans to assess blood flow to the uterus at around 24 weeks.
- Previous late miscarriage or premature labour and delivery: serial ultrasound assessment of the length of the cervix to predict the likelihood of recurrence and individualise management.

Third Trimester

You will be seen quite frequently (usually every two weeks from 28 weeks and weekly from 36 weeks) in this last part of pregnancy for blood pressure and urine checks and examination of your baby. Raised blood pressure (see Pre-eclampsia, page 48) and impaired glucose metabolism are two of the most common problems of the third trimester.

Glucose Testing

Some women have diabetes before they get pregnant and are usually under the care of a diabetes team already. 'Gestational diabetes', however, occurs only during pregnancy and is a relatively common condition which can potentially affect how well the mother feels and the growth of her baby (page 49). As with many antenatal tests, different units offer different forms of testing for this condition. Some screen all women, usually at between 26 and 30 weeks' gestation. Others offer a selective screening policy, such as screening only women with certain risk factors like a family history of diabetes.

The test involves drinking a sugary drink and checking your blood sugar levels at a particular time later (usually one to two hours).

Other Tests

Some women will need closer surveillance in the last trimester, especially if they appear to be developing any complication. Some of the more common third trimester problems are listed below:

- Raised blood pressure: additional blood and urine tests may be required.
- Concerns about fetal growth: additional scans and blood flow (Doppler) ultrasound examination may be offered.
- Preterm rupture of membranes: vaginal and perineal swabs for infective causes such as Group B streptococcus are usually recommended.

RELATIVELY COMMON MEDICAL PROBLEMS

Pre-eclampsia

It is usual for blood pressure to rise slightly in the third trimester. In about 10 per cent of women this rise is quite marked and needs close monitoring, usually with weekly out-patient checks, and possibly the use of antihypertensive medication. This is a condition called pregnancy-induced hypertension. In a small minority of women (1 to 2 per cent), the blood pressure elevation is associated with protein excretion in your urine and/or swelling or fluid retention in your legs, fingers and face, and this condition is called pre-eclampsia. When your midwife checks your blood pressure and dip-tests your urine at each check-up, this is the condition she is looking out for. Pre-eclampsia usually occurs in the third trimester but can occur earlier in some women. Whenever it is suspected, women are referred to an obstetrician who will assess them and recommend the necessary surveillance and management.

The 'cure' for pre-eclampsia is delivery, and in early onset or severe cases this may need to be done prematurely and/or by Caesarean section. However, most cases are mild and if you are towards the end of your pregnancy and your blood pressure continues to rise, or stays high (usually 140/90 or above), it is likely that induction of labour will be recommended to you in order to expedite delivery.

Usually the rise in blood pressure occurs fairly gradually and there is sufficient time to monitor progression and investigate on an outpatient basis. Occasionally pre-eclampsia can develop very quickly, so if you know you have a tendency towards high blood pressure, **call your hospital if you develop any of the following:**

- **a bad headache that doesn't respond to simple pain killers**
- **sudden swelling of your face, fingers and legs**
- **seeing spots or flashing lights in front of your eyes or blurred vision**
- **pain in your upper tummy, just below your ribcage on the right hand side**

You will be reviewed promptly rather than having to wait for another week or so until your routine check-up is due. Pre-eclampsia rarely causes problems if its signs and symptoms are reported early and appropriate investigations and management plans carried out without delay.

Gestational Diabetes

This is a condition when the blood sugar level rises because there is insufficient insulin for its metabolism. It occurs in 1 to 2 per cent of all pregnancies in the UK, but the prevalence is much greater in women from certain ethnic minority groups. It is largely, although not exclusively, a third trimester phenomenon and as such is very distinct from pre-existing diabetes i.e. when the woman has known that she has diabetes mellitus for a long time before getting pregnant and has been taking tablets or insulin to control her blood sugar levels for some time.

Gestational diabetes develops during pregnancy and disappears after delivery and is therefore a temporary condition. Maternity Units vary in the way that they screen for this condition, but the national recommendations are that women at risk of developing gestational diabetes have a 'glucose challenge test' where they drink a set measure of a sugary drink, such as Lucozade, and after a fixed time interval (usually one or two hours) a blood test is taken.

If you screen positive, you are considered to have gestational diabetes and are referred for joint care in a hospital-based Antenatal Clinic with a Diabetes Centre.

Treatment in most cases is with a special diet and you will need to use a pocket-sized home monitoring device to measure your blood sugar levels at certain points during the day. Most women with gestational diabetes can control their blood sugar levels with diet alone, but a small minority require insulin injections which they are taught to give to themselves. Although this might sound troublesome and may not be what you want to be spending time on in the last few weeks of your pregnancy, it very rarely causes difficulty and the Diabetes Team (which will include a dietitian, a midwife and a doctor) provide excellent support and training for this.

You will also have extra scans in pregnancy if you develop gestational diabetes as occasionally babies can grow rather bigger than average. Women with poorly controlled gestational diabetes may need to be induced a week or two before their due date (see page 99).

Placenta Praevia

The placenta is usually sited towards the top and back of the uterus. At the routine 20-week scan, 15 per cent of women are found to have a placenta that is lying low and close to the cervix. At this stage it does not necessarily mean you have a placenta praevia; you simply need to be scanned again in the third trimester, usually between 32 and 34 weeks' gestation. In the vast majority of women, the placenta will 'move up' as the uterus grows, and will therefore not be likely to cause bleeding or an obstruction to the labour. In about 1 per cent of pregnancies, this third trimester scan will reveal that the placenta is partially (or occasionally even completely) covering the cervix, and this is a placenta praevia.

Clearly this may cause vaginal bleeding, in which case you may need to be hospitalised. Delivery in these cases is always by Caesarean section. There is absolutely nothing you can do to prevent or cure this condition but be thankful that it can be diagnosed with great certainty nowadays, and that when your obstetrician knows about this condition, provisions will be made for you to deliver in the safest place possible for both you and your baby.

Most healthy women have uncomplicated pregnancies and the investigations that are carried out in the antenatal period are seen as straightforward and routine. However, some women will have unexpected results and complications, and the key to good clinical management is regular antenatal check-ups and picking up and acting upon early warning signs. Remember, if midwives and obstetricians get this bit right, you are more likely to go into the labour and delivery phase well-informed and as healthy as possible, and that undoubtedly has a beneficial effect upon you and your baby.

CHAPTER 4

work issues

You have discovered you are pregnant. Let's say you are in your late twenties or early thirties and have worked for the same company for the last eight years – you're thrilled about the baby but you also love your job!

There are three issues to be confronted:

- When are you going to tell them you are pregnant?
- When is the best time to give up work?
- When is a realistic time to return?

WHEN TO TELL WORK YOU ARE PREGNANT

It is only fair to let your boss know as soon as possible so she or he has time to plan ahead and work out cover arrangements for you. The problem is, you probably won't want to tempt fate and announce your good news until you know that your pregnancy is stable. How many weeks pregnant you are is calculated from the first day of your last period (see page 8). Most women can relax when they reach 13 weeks, and this would seem to be a good time to tell people at work.

The downside to this plan is that if you have been throwing up and feeling like death, none of your work colleagues will have known why (unless they guessed) so may not have been as sympathetic as they would have been otherwise. By the time you tell them you are pregnant you will be starting to feel much better.

At this stage you will also need to find out how many weeks' paid leave you are entitled to and what sort of deal your boss is prepared to give you. This obviously varies in individual cases and between companies, but statutory pregnancy leave is now 26 weeks. During this leave, as long as you are not working, you will be entitled to Statutory Maternity Pay (SMP), which is paid by your employer. In order for this to happen, you need a form – Mat B1 (confirming your estimated date of delivery, EDD) – but this can't be collected from your GP until you are 20 weeks pregnant.

WHEN TO GIVE UP WORK

Most career women won't believe this, but it is best for both you and your baby if you give up work when you are 34 weeks pregnant. That is six weeks before your baby is due.

I can hear the objections:

- Good grief! That's ridiculous! I'm feeling absolutely fine. What on earth is the point of lying around at home for six weeks (or even eight weeks as first babies are 'always late')?

- What on earth am I going to do with the time?
- I shall get dreadfully bored and depressed.
- How stupid to use up all my maternity leave before the baby is born. It's obviously much better to work as late as possible, as apart from anything else I'll have more time afterwards to be with my baby.
- Anyway, it's completely out of the question because my boss has three children and with each pregnancy she was in her office until the head crowned and back at her desk two weeks later.

But of the thousands of pregnant women I have seen, nearly *everyone* – be she a doctor, a teacher, a secretary, a lawyer, a banker or someone who runs her own business – will tell the same story. Unbelievable as it may sound beforehand, **when you reach 34 weeks you start losing interest in your work** so even going to work becomes an effort. **This is especially relevant if you work very long hours and/or have to make quick decisions.**

(Incidentally, if you are a pilot, you are not allowed to fly a plane after 28 weeks, which is interesting…)

If it is possible, it is better to divide up your maternity leave, and perhaps add on some holiday time, so that you finish earlier and go back earlier. **Under no circumstances agree to work beyond 36 weeks, which is four weeks before your baby is due.**

These are some of the reasons:

- First babies are *not* always late, in spite of what your girlfriends tell you. From my figures, 50 per cent are late, 25 per cent are born on time and 25 per cent are born early.

This means that if you are working until 38 weeks, it is quite possible you may have your baby the day you are due to leave work. Apart from the obvious lack of preparation that would result from this, are you really prepared to risk your waters breaking during a meeting or when you are seeing a client?

- The baby you are carrying is more important to you than almost anything else – this goes without saying. Although he has not yet been born, he is still very much there. You want to give him the best care in pregnancy, just as you will want to make sure that he is looked after properly when he has been born.

- He is absolutely dependent on you now, and that means he needs you to slow down and take a rest during the day at the end of your pregnancy. Rest increases blood flow to your baby: if a baby is thought to be small for dates many obstetricians will put mothers on bed-rest to help their baby grow. (You may have noticed how dramatically your baby grows when you spend a couple of weeks sitting around a poolside on holiday.) It is unlikely that your place of work will be equipped with a bed to enable you to do this, which is another reason for not working beyond 34 weeks. Another indication for bed-rest is when a mother's blood pressure is up – sometimes it comes down to a normal level simply if the woman stays in bed. Raised blood pressure in a pregnant woman is always taken seriously (see Pre-eclampsia, page 48).

- Surveys show that women who work in high-pressure jobs beyond 35 weeks of pregnancy are more likely to have early babies and more complications, such as high blood pressure. This is confirmed by the women I see!

- Giving up work and having a baby are both major life events. Life events are stressful, even when they are pleasurable. The task of adjusting to two life events in a short space of time increases the risk of stress-related disorders. It doesn't take a genius to see that it's sensible to try and separate these two life events by more than a week or so.

- Something very odd happens to women in pregnancy – they are likely to lose their self-confidence, their memory (have you noticed that you already seem to be making rather a lot of lists?) and their ability to make decisions. On top of all this, many women will find themselves bursting into tears (so embarrassing) for no real reason. These changes are not within our control any more than PMT changes are – the difference is that they become more marked as pregnancy progresses, whereas at least PMT is cyclical.

- Another even odder change is that you will find you start to become interested in baby clothes and – to your horror – notice you have begun to look into other people's prams (yes, even you). This growing interest in babies is called primary maternal preoccupation, and it is nature's way of making sure that women are in an appropriate state of mind to care for their baby when he is born – another reason why work becomes less interesting.

- Getting into the siesta habit is something you will need to do when you have had your baby – you are probably going to be more sleep-deprived then than you can ever imagine, and if you are unable to take a nap during the afternoon you will have a problem.

- It is difficult to imagine how physically incapacitated you may become at the end of your pregnancy, especially if you have put on more weight than the books describe. Getting in and out of a car can be difficult enough, let alone putting on your tights.

- You are much more likely to enjoy your pregnancy and the first few months with your baby if you acknowledge the physiological and psychological changes in you now, and are prepared for the changes to come. Labour is arduous enough without going into it already exhausted. The emotional impact of your first baby is greater than any woman can imagine beforehand and you really do not want to be so swamped by these events that you don't enjoy your baby. You certainly don't want to collapse with exhaustion when he is three or four months old – and you are shortly expected back at work.

COPING WITH WORK AND PREGNANCY

Let's assume you are conscientious and want to do your job as well as possible and continue working the hours you are paid for. At the same time you have to try and find a balance so you don't end up so exhausted that your doctor puts you on compulsory bed-rest. This means being realistic about the changes that will automatically happen to you as your pregnancy progresses, as well as the possible physical symptoms you might experience. Rather than just carrying on as though nothing has happened, coping with work successfully will be easier if you plan ahead. Unfortunately, even women with the strongest willpower can't prevent the physical side-effects of pregnancy, such as nausea, fatigue or sometimes a complication such as a rise in blood pressure. If you are proactive, allowing for these possible changes and actually planning your workload before you go on maternity leave, hopefully you will not become stressed.

It will help if you are sensitive to the fact that what may be the most exciting and dramatic news to you isn't necessarily particularly thrilling for the people you work with. In fact, most people's initial private thought is, 'Oh God, couldn't she have timed things better – how am I going to cope with all her work at that particularly busy time of year?' If you sense a somewhat dismissive reaction, don't feel hurt and brood. And once your office knows the news, don't go on about it! Incidentally, only you (and presumably your obstetrician and the radiographer) will be able to recognise a baby from the ultrasound Polaroid.

You will need to accept that you will slow down during pregnancy and lose a little of your buzz. The biggest practical problem for working women who are pregnant is getting enough rest. From 28 weeks, it is important for you and your baby if you can lie down for an hour at some time during the day, because when you lie down, there is an increase of blood flow to the placenta, which in turn will help your baby grow. Lying down at some stage during the day will also reduce your chances of getting low backache and may help prevent your blood pressure going up. Some offices may have a rest-room which you can use during your lunch hour – if this is a possibility, use it. *If you can find the confidence to do this, you will be establishing a precedent for future pregnant women!* Make it clear that you are not lying down during the day because you are a wimp and making a fuss about being pregnant – you are lying down so that the blood supply to the placenta is increased, which is in the interests of your baby. For those of you with absolutely nowhere to lie down during the day, go straight to bed for an hour when you get home.

Look ahead in your diary and write in how many weeks pregnant you will be each week. Try to make sure that you don't have to sit or stand for long periods, as when you are more than 28 weeks pregnant you will find you need to alter your position frequently. After 32 weeks, don't commit yourself to long car journeys (let alone air flights). Also, be very careful that you don't agree to projects with vital deadlines after this stage, and avoid taking on work that culminates in you having to give a mega presentation just before you are due to go on maternity leave. The chances are that you will not be up to your usual standard, and it might be worth bearing in mind that after 30 weeks most women sleep badly at night!

If you are attending a long meeting, find out where the loo is first as you will notice that your bladder seems to be very small. Check that your chair is at the correct height for your desk, and if you spend most of your day at a computer, get up every two hours and walk around. If your job involves lifting, remember to bend your knees and keep your back straight as you do so – your lower back is very vulnerable during pregnancy (see page 121). You will find that you may not be able to skip meals as before – lunch will be imperative, and you might need to allow time for this, especially if you have been used to an emergency lunch of a chocolate bar in the early afternoon.

When you are pregnant you cannot walk as fast as you normally do, so you will need to allow more time for the walk from the train or bus. Most women say that it is not so much their actual work that is stressful, but the problem of a long journey getting there, especially if it involves travelling by public transport. You may have an acute sense of smell, so standing in a crowded train is even more unpleasant than usual. If you feel or are being sick in the early weeks, there is also a serious problem of how to manage the journey without throwing up. Morning sickness usually passes at around the 14-week mark, but for some unlucky women it can continue for much longer (see page 12).

If you are used to putting in long hours, when you reach 28 weeks, try and have a good think about your working week, and see if there is any possibility of working from home one day. And if you think this is feasible, discuss the practicalities with your boss. An alternative option may be to cut back your hours now, and for the first few months when you return.

It is only fair to you, your baby (and your boss!) to be realistic about your social life outside work and curtail some of your evening activities. It may be a good idea to set priorities in your social life – to be honest it is probably a good idea to instate a rule that you never go out two nights running. You really won't feel like working a full day, nipping into the supermarket on your way home, having a quick swim and then having friends for supper! Similarly it's best to make sure that your weekends don't consist of looking at new flats or houses, then a shopping session followed by visiting your parents. At the risk of sounding really boring, your weekend is when you are able to, and should, have a nap in the afternoon – especially important if you are not able to lie down during the week.

WHEN IS THE BEST TIME TO GO BACK TO WORK?

With any luck, when your baby is about 14–16 weeks he will be sleeping through the night. At this time, hopefully you should feel much less tired than you did beforehand. (Most women feel most tired when their baby is 10 weeks old.) Returning to work earlier than 16 weeks is possible, but tough. If you are lucky enough to be able to dictate when you will return to work (as opposed to having no choice because you have a mortgage to pay) the optimal time seems to be when your baby is around five to six months. And even then, you won't want to leave him, so if you are able to negotiate returning for three or four days a week, that would be even better.

Longer maternity leave has meant that many women now don't have to return to work until much later than this, but from my experience, women find it more difficult to return to work when their baby is older than six months. There are two possible reasons for this.

Firstly, babies develop something called separation anxiety at around six to seven months. This is totally normal, but it means they cling to you when strangers enter the house and cry when you leave the room. (This can be quite irritating, as you find that you can't even go to the loo without taking your baby with you.) It doesn't mean you have already done something wrong on the mothering front – it is normal child development. But it makes leaving your baby to go to work more emotionally draining for you.

The other reason is more difficult to state clearly. Many women find that as they become immersed in motherhood, their life-focus becomes entirely baby-orientated. This, coupled with trying to leave a tearful, clingy baby, makes going back to work a very unattractive prospect.

Making realistic, sensible decisions about your working life will be best in the long run for both you and your baby. In the next chapter we will look at some of the practical steps you can take to make sure you are well organised for the new arrival.

CHAPTER 5

getting organised

This chapter is about doing some constructive planning and preparation. If you can start to get organised now, it will mean that you will also start to focus on what life will be like when you actually come home with your baby. **This is the really important bit!** Try very hard not to focus only on the birth – otherwise you are more likely to be knocked sideways after your baby is born. So in this bit you are thinking way beyond the birth and focusing on getting ready for when you come home with your new baby.

I know many of you will find it almost impossible to believe that you will be lucky enough to come home with a healthy baby. It's a concept that's really difficult to handle – and in the same way, many women in my antenatal classes find the feeding class difficult to take in ('Will this really be me who comes home with a normal baby and have to feed it?'). You may feel so worried about the birth, you reckon if you can survive that, the baby will be a breeze. You might also irrationally feel that if you buy all the gear beforehand, this will tempt fate and something will go horribly wrong. But even if you want to postpone getting stuff delivered until after your baby has been born, you still need to buy certain items of equipment, and think about what he will sleep in and where you will change him and so on.

BABY GEAR AND EQUIPMENT

This can seem really daunting! But you usually don't need as much as you think and some of the equipment is used for only a few months. Your baby won't know if it is new or second-hand, so if you have friends or relatives who offer to lend you anything, accept with gratitude! Don't get into the mindset that your baby will think you are a second-rate mother if you borrow stuff. Try and avoid buying any expensive furniture that has a nursery decoration on, such as yellow and brown bunnies – you really won't want to keep it in your child's room for the next 10 years so it's better to buy furniture that will still work as your baby grows up.

It's a mistake to leave everything to the last minute! ('Well, when I give up work at 34 weeks we'll spend Saturday morning in John Lewis or Mothercare and perhaps nip over to IKEA.') The process of buying all the kit is unlikely to be as simple as you think and there is no way you will be able to cope with the IKEA nightmare as well. Apart from the fact that you may not be in a fit state to survive a morning of standing and trying to make decisions, some items may well have to be ordered and can take up to 10 weeks to arrive. Most of the nursery gear will be self-assembly – and you know what that means.

Gear for You

The following need to be bought early, as you will use them at the end of pregnancy as well as when you come home.

Extra Pillows and/or a V-shaped Pillow

Extra pillows will help you get into a comfortable position to sleep at the end of pregnancy (see page 154). Later on, you will probably use one or two pillows to lie your baby on when you are feeding him. If you have a family history of allergies, you may want to avoid feather pillows near your baby. A V-shaped pillow is something you will find useful forever!

Mattress Cover

If you don't already have one, a fitted cotton padded mattress cover (try John Lewis or M&S) is best, as it will protect your mattress from the inevitable baby sick and worse. And when you are 37 weeks pregnant, it will be thick enough for you not to notice a bin liner you can put under your side of the bed, which will protect your mattress if your waters break in bed (see Chapter 11).

Cotton Nightshirts

You'll find it useful to have three cotton nightshirts with buttons down the front. These are sometimes incredibly difficult to find, which is why they are on the 'buy early' list. Try online maternity shops, nightwear suppliers, Mothercare and M&S. You will spend some or all of labour in your own nightdress, and even if you sleep in the buff normally, when you return home you absolutely won't want to be padding round with a sanitary pad and a bra and no cover-up. You will find it best if they are cotton, short-sleeved, knee-length, not see-through and with buttons opening well down to below your breasts.

Low Nursing Chair

Traditional nursing chairs have low seats – 30–40 cm (12–14 inches) from the floor – and no arms. This design enables a mother to breast- (or bottle-) feed her baby without having to bend forwards – so she is in a comfortable position and less likely to strain her upper back. An upright kitchen chair is terribly uncomfortable in the middle of the night! You don't have to buy one specifically, but it's worth asking your parents if they have an old nursing chair stored in their loft. Otherwise, if you have nothing suitable, a low upholstered bedroom-type chair without arms and usually found in a department store would work.

Two or Three Nursing Bras (see page 143)

Disposable Breast Pads

Many women find that they leak milk from their breasts between feeds, and from the breast they are not feeding from during a feed. The pads will keep your bra (and top clothes) dry.

Sanitary/Maternity Pads

It is normal to bleed quite heavily from where the placenta was attached to the uterus (lochia) directly after your baby has been born. Even if you have a Caesarean section, you should not (and will not want to) use tampons.

Gear for Your Baby

Baby Car Seat

The law now states that a baby can't travel in a car without being in a car seat, so this is vital equipment. Unfortunately, not all car seats fit all cars, so you need to arrange a trip with your husband (and your car!) to buy one before you are 34 weeks pregnant. It is helpful if your husband goes with you, as he will be responsible for getting your baby safely in the car when he collects you both from hospital – you may not be able to stand for long enough to do so. It probably isn't necessary to buy a car seat that fits onto wheels – in any case, most babies seem happier wheeled around a shop lying flat in a pram, which is stored in the boot of your car. Most mothers say that the easiest (and cheapest) first car seat is a carry in/carry out one fixed into position by your own car seat belts, rather than a complicated travel system involving an isofix. Most baby-gear shops (including very large Mothercare branches) will tell you which car seats are suitable for your car and actually show you how to fix your car seat belt around it. Nothing is as easy as it looks if you haven't done it before.

Moses Basket or Something Similar

For the first few months, your baby will probably sleep with you in your bedroom (see page 75). Most parents borrow or buy a Moses basket or a light pram top. If you live in a flat and your bedroom is on the same floor as your sitting room, it's OK for your baby to sleep in his pram (as long as it's flat). But if your bedroom is upstairs, you won't want to carry the pram, or even just the pram top, up and down the stairs more than necessary.

Pram

Buying the right pram can seem as complicated as buying the right car. If you go with your partner to have a look at what's on offer it's likely to take a very long time, as he will get very enthused... There are no prams that mothers constantly rate as the best – but your young baby must be able to sleep completely flat. The pram you go for is a personal decision, depending very much on:

- the entrance to your house – will you have to carry it up to your front door and, if so, is it light enough?
- whether you plan to have another baby quickly – do you need a pram that will take a toddler as well as a baby?
- the layout of your house
- your budget

If you are going to buy a new pram, start looking into this very early on and go to a shop where you can actually try out the assembly and wheel various models around.

Nursery Gear

Changing table or chest of drawers with changing mat
This is essential for endless nappy changing, in spite of whoever might tell you to use the floor! Check that this comes up to the **height of your waist** so you are not leaning forwards when you change your baby because this will give you low backache. It is much better to buy something with drawers or a cupboard for storing clothes, so you can keep it as a piece of nursery furniture long after your baby is out of nappies. A changing trolley with open shelves underneath will not be useful when your baby is on his feet, as he will unpack everything from the shelves...

Plastic changing mat

If your bedroom is upstairs, you might think about buying two of these and keeping one downstairs. This will save you having to stagger upstairs every time you change his nappy. In any case, they are also useful for your baby to lie on without a nappy and have a kick in the evening. The second mat could be a foldable portable one, which you can use not only at home, but stick in your changing bag (see page 71) when you go out.

Plug-in baby monitor

These are available from all baby shops, and allow you to hear your baby cry if he is in a different room to you – essential for your peace of mind.

Pack of muslins

These are for mopping up sick and some of you will use them to cover your baby's changing mat. You will need several muslins (or terry nappies or small towels) to go on top of the changing mat, partially to absorb baby pee when you change him, and partially to prevent him having to lie on cold plastic. The reason you need several is because they will usually go straight into the washing machine after use.

First size disposable nappies (2–5 kg, 4–11 lb) and nappy sacks

Even if you choose to use washable nappies for your baby in the long term, for the first few weeks baby poo can be very runny and very frequent! You may find you go through around 10 nappies a day with a new baby. Not everyone agrees on which nappies are the best, so buy two or three different brands and then decide which is right for you.

Bowl for warm water

If your changing table is not near running water, you will have to wash your baby's bottom in water carried in a bowl to the changing mat.

Large cotton wool balls

You will use these to wash a dirty bottom – make sure you don't get a cotton wool pleat that you need two hands to tear off as you will need one of your hands to hold your baby's legs.

Zinc and castor oil cream or Sudocrem

Both are barrier creams to protect your baby's bottom. Zinc and castor oil cream (from any chemist) is cheaper, but Sudocrem has a healing property, so you will tend to use it if your baby has a hint of a sore bottom.

Baby bath or something similar

There are many different types on the market, and all claim to make bath-time easier. But they are not absolutely essential if you are short of space, as it is possible (but difficult) to bath your baby in your sink or a big bath – preferably with your partner in it as well. If you can borrow a baby bath, do so.

Baby bath solution, baby soap (Simple soap) or aqueous cream

Two soft towels for the baby's use only

You don't have to buy special baby towels, but they need to be earmarked for your baby only. In the early days, especially before his cord has dropped off, it's best not to dry him with towels that might harbour someone else's bacteria.

Small sponge for washing your baby

Baby nail scissors, emery board or nail clippers
Some babies have very long fingernails – use what you find easiest to trim them with.

Baby hairbrush
And some babies have masses of hair!

Car window sun-screener (especially in spring)
Babies hate bright sun in their eyes.

Portable changing bag
Use anything that will take nappies, bottom-cleaning equipment, a change of baby clothes and possibly a bottle and formula milk. This means you can visit people with all your necessary baby gear.

Bouncing cradle
This is a valuable piece of equipment if you can find a good one. Unlike car seats, they are comfortable for your baby, and allow him to sit or lie at various angles. Ideally, you need one that you can rock your baby to sleep in (while you are trying to have supper) but will also sit him up slightly so he can see what is going on when he is awake and alert. If you can't find anything suitable, ring Babylist (020 7371 5145) who stock a very good cradle that is not available in the usual department stores.

Two or three swaddling sheets (sometimes called receiving sheets)
What on earth are these? See page 74.

Three fitted bottom sheets for crib/Moses basket and pram
You won't need top sheets, as your baby will be swaddled.

Three blankets for crib/Moses basket and pram
Possibly one wool and two cotton cellular.

Plastic mattress sheet (if your mattress is borrowed and not already covered with one)

Four to six cotton vests
Choose the over-the-head type. It doesn't matter if they don't have crutch poppers – in fact, for a new baby who doesn't move very much, you might find the extra poppers a nuisance when you've already undone all the poppers on a babygro.

Four to six nightgowns and/or babygros
Nightgowns make nappy changing very much easier (especially in the night) but you will sort out what works best for you.

Cardigans and socks

Bonnet
Babies lose most of their body heat through their head – even if yours is an (English) summer baby, he will need a bonnet.

Bibs
You may not like the look of bibs, but buy a pack of inexpensive soft ones. Some babies are remarkably messy when feeding and many babies vomit small (or large) amounts of milk after a feed. You will

be anxious not to add anything more than necessary to your large pile of washing.

Dummies!

Dummies often evoke tut-tuttings, as some people think that if a baby uses a dummy, he will be plugged in for the following four years or so. This is absolutely not true. Although not all babies need one, a dummy can be a great help to an unsettled or 'sucky' baby for the first few months. You can buy specific orthodontic newborn dummies (usually described as 0–4 months) which have an extra small teat. A dummy will not ruin your baby's future tooth formation (ask any orthodontist) as long as they are discarded early. When your baby is around four to five months old, he will be able to find his own fingers or thumb if he needs to, or will have learnt other self-soothing skills, so the dummy can be discarded.

Later On, When Baby is in his Own Room

Side light with low-wattage bulb or night light

This is necessary for trying to settle or feed your baby in the night, without waking him up by putting on a full light. Later on, a night light may be necessary to find dropped dummies.

Heater with thermostatic control for winter babies

Your baby needs to sleep in a room where the temperature is reasonably constant – around 18°C.

Fan for summer babies

You can guarantee there will be a shortage of fans during an unexpected heat wave. Homebase supply a good range of quiet floor-standing fans.

I don't think you need blackout blinds! They are an unnecessary expense, and when you go to stay with other people, it's unlikely that they will have them. This can leave you with the problem of a baby who can't settle for a daytime sleep.

And finally…

These days, you don't need to wash new stuff before using it for your baby. Also, friends can be extremely generous when it comes to a new baby, so don't unpack anything you buy that can be changed, and keep the receipts.

SWADDLING

Small babies need, and like, to be swaddled. It is an ancient practice. When a baby is lying on his back, swaddling will contain his normal startle reflex, which is when his arms jerk upwards in response to a noise or slight movement, and wakes and unsettles him. It also makes him feel secure, so he will sleep better. We now know that babies must sleep on their backs – cot deaths have halved since mothers have been advised to put babies to sleep on their back rather than on their tummy. You might be told that swaddling a baby increases the risk of cot death – statistically this is not true, but nevertheless, take care your baby doesn't overheat.

Buying (or Making) a Swaddling Sheet

In an ideal world, it's best to make your own if you can and have the time. You need a sheet measuring approximately 110 cm by 85 cm. This must be cotton (or winceyette) material. If you want to buy a ready-made one, it doesn't need to have a Velcro fastening, and shouldn't be made out of stretchy material. Stretchy material won't contain your baby properly, and if it is a double fabric, there is the danger of him overheating.

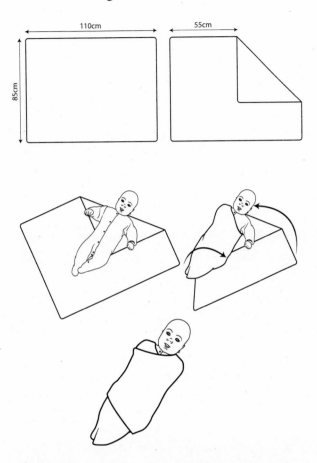

WHERE WILL THE BABY SLEEP?

In spite of what you might decide before your baby is born, nearly all new parents feel most comfortable with their new baby sleeping in their bedroom – and, as it happens, the Foundation for the Study of Infant Deaths recommends your baby sleeps in your bedroom (with you!). (You will be given a leaflet about cot deaths, which will make you extremely anxious.) Your baby can sleep in a Moses basket, a pram top or in a pram (or, actually, in a large drawer!) next, or near, to your bed. As new mothers don't generally feel comfortable being separated from their babies, and as he will need to be fed during the night, this seems the obvious place for him to be. So the best plan (if your bedroom is big enough) is to assume he will sleep in the same room as you initially, and then to see how it goes.

WILL I BREASTFEED?

Everyone knows that breast milk is best for babies – after all, nature has had several million years to get it perfect. But babies will also thrive perfectly satisfactorily on formula milk if necessary. It has to be said that no-one can tell by looking at a group of children (or university students) which were breastfed and which were bottle-fed.

Your milk doesn't 'come in' until three or four days after birth, and before that your breasts produce a small amount of cloudy yellow fluid called colostrum. This is very important for your baby – it is full of your antibodies, which give him protection against infections, as well as other 'goodies' – and there is absolutely no substitute. Bearing this in mind, it would seem sensible to plan to start off at least by giving your baby your precious colostrum, and simply see how breastfeeding goes from there. For the majority of women, this approach works well.

Even if you plan to breastfeed, you will need to buy:

- one bottle and first-size teat
- some sort of newborn formula milk (small ready-made cartons are useful as you don't need to add cooled boiled water)

Buying the above is a precaution against coming home to a middle-of-the-night crisis with a day-old, screaming and apparently starving baby, who, having taken colostrum satisfactorily in hospital, appears to have forgotten how to suckle.

If you plan to bottle feed from the start, you will need to buy:

- six bottles
- six teats
- a bottle brush
- a steriliser
- a plastic jug
- a plastic knife
- sterilising solution or tablets

I have been struck by the number of women who have said to me during their antenatal classes that they **definitely don't want to breastfeed,** but having started off with giving their baby colostrum, go on to breastfeed him quite happily for several months! Conversely, I have come across many women who are determined to breastfeed, but sadly find it terribly difficult so their baby needs formula milk in order to thrive. For the majority of women, breastfeeding goes well, and apart from being the best option, it is eventually the easiest. But the most important concern is that your baby gets food – breast or bottle. Like labour, you simply don't know how straightforward things are going to be – so just keep an open mind.

I am not an expert on breast- or bottle-feeding. The best book on the subject is *What to Expect When You're Breast-feeding...and What If You Can't* by Clare Byam-Cook, published by Vermilion (see page 247).

ORGANISING SOMEONE TO LOOK AFTER YOU

Provided there are no problems, you will be sent home extremely soon after delivery – between six and twenty-four hours following a straightforward vaginal birth, and between twenty-four hours and three days after a Caesarean section. You will need someone around to help you. This is really important – don't underestimate how vulnerable and spaced out you will feel, however capable you are normally. It will be doubly important if you have a Caesarean section because you won't be able to stand for long periods of time. And of course it may be impossible to avoid standing for long periods when you are trying to calm an unsettled baby. With any luck, your husband will be able to be with you for the first day or two – and he is nearly always your best choice of helper in the early days. Generally speaking, most new parents tell me that it was really good having the first couple of days together, quietly on their own with their baby, rather than arriving home to find a third person waiting in the kitchen.

You should plan to spend the first week in your night gear, in or around your bed, with your baby beside you. This is where you need to be – it is your 'lying-in' period, and essential in order for you to recover physically, start to establish breastfeeding and generally get to know and fall into step with your baby. You will also need to adjust quietly not only to your wonderful baby, but to the daunting realisation that he is totally dependent on you – and at a time when you will not be feeling exactly robust yourself.

You will need to eat proper meals (obviously) but will find that it is difficult to organise the shopping and preparation of food at the same time as caring for a new baby, not to mention keeping the house clean. Just how you arrange someone else to come and give you a hand with all this will depend on how much time your partner can take off. Statutory paternity leave is two weeks, but in practice, many men can't manage to escape from work pressures for as long as this (especially if they are self-employed) so it's probably important to have a realistic discussion with him well beforehand. This is obviously especially important if your mother has offered to help, but doesn't live nearby, so may have no alternative but to stay with you for a few days.

Most women will enlist extra help in the form of a mother, mother-in-law or perhaps a sister. To be honest, if you are lucky enough to have a mother or mother-in-law who you get on with and who is willing to help, you are very lucky. The big difference between your own family helping out and employing someone else (see overleaf) is that your own mother loves you and will love your baby. This can only be good news for both of you. You really don't have to have a professional to 'teach' you how to care for your baby – babies are pretty parent-proof and you will actually manage the early weeks with the help of your community midwife and your health visitor.

I talk to countless women about all this, and, of course, some of you have mothers who for various reasons are not suitable ('don't do babies'), are needed elsewhere to care for a sick relative, are not well themselves or simply unavailable for several other reasons. When I say, 'Do you get on with your mother-in-law, and is she a possibility?' you frequently reply, 'Oh yes, we get on really well, and she lives very near but she's a high-powered something-or-other and couldn't possibly take the time off.' Usually, if they actually approach their mother-in-law, she is quite delighted to help, and of course can fix to take time off, but hadn't dare suggest it in case of being thought pushy or intrusive. Have a discussion with your partner as soon as you can and work out what would seem to be the best option for you both. But bear in mind that if you have working mothers, as many of you will, they will need to be asked sooner rather than later so they can sort out their diaries.

Other Options to Consider

You may be in the difficult position of having no family nearby and a husband who can only take a couple of days off, but you feel you really won't be able to cope with (or afford) professional help. You may also be the sort of woman who reads the above paragraph with horror – you don't get on with your mother, you absolutely don't get on with your mother-in-law, and in any case you like to be on your own! If you fall into this group, perhaps you could consider employing someone simply to clean the house for you, or if you already have someone, asking if she could do a couple of extra hours a week. Do you have a girlfriend who might be able to help you out for a week or two?

Professional Help

Some of you, whatever the reason, will have decided that you want professional help such as a maternity nurse or a doula (see below). It may be that you are expected back at work very soon, or are expecting twins. Even if you are planning to return to work full-time and engage a live-in nanny, it's usually best to wait until you have had your baby before finding the right nanny (see page 84). In the early weeks, most women opting for professional help will go for a maternity nurse or (increasingly) a doula.

Maternity Nurses

This is the most expensive option you can go for – currently between £700 and £900 a week. Most maternity nurses will live with you, so there is the added cost of board and food. A few women will find that their parents offer to pay, but even so, only a handful of families can consider this. Nevertheless, I have included some information below for the minority of you that will use one.

What is She?

A maternity nurse may have trained as a midwife or nurse or possibly a nanny. Some may have had specific maternity nurse training. A few older maternity nurses have had no formal training but simply years of experience looking after babies, and some may have had children of their own. Their job is to support you and to help and teach you to look after your baby, so you will gain confidence. The main advantage is that they will also help in the night, so a new mother has the bonus of being able to get a bit more sleep.

Where Do You Find One?

From my experience, it is always preferable (though a heavy added expense) to go through a specialist agency, rather than just by word of mouth or through an advertisement in the paper. Firstly, agencies are extremely careful and conscientious about checking references. Secondly, they will draw up a contract, and if there is a hitch – such as the nurse becoming ill as she is due to start with you or you finding that you both don't get on when she has started – it is the agency's responsibility (rather than yours) to sort things out. The same applies if your baby arrives unexpectedly early – you won't be in any condition to find an emergency replacement, and agencies are usually good at finding someone on a short-term basis if necessary.

How Long Will I Need Her?

Traditionally, maternity nurses were employed for four weeks – which is why they are sometimes called a monthly nurse. But the vast majority of women report back to me that three weeks is quite long enough – unless you have an extremely large home! I would say that under normal circumstances, ten days to three weeks is fine. Paradoxically, I've noticed that when we see mothers and babies at postnatal classes, the longer women have had a maternity nurse, the less confident they are handling their own baby.

Deciding on a starting date for her is difficult, as you don't know exactly when your baby will arrive – but this is a common problem. On the whole, it usually works best to book her start date for a week or so after your EDD – but this obviously depends on individual circumstances.

If your baby arrives unexpectedly early, it is usually possible to find a maternity nurse who is free for a few days between bookings. Incidentally, this is also an option if you are in two minds about whether you want or can afford to hire professional help. Similarly, some women find that they are fine for the first four weeks or so, then it gradually transpires that they have a difficult baby and need a week's help later, when they are really sleep deprived. An agency nearly always manages to find someone who is free at short notice for an emergency bale-out.

How Do I Find the Right One for Me?

If your maternity nurse will be living in your home, it's important that you meet up with her before you engage her. This will give you both an opportunity to see if the chemistry between you is right and have a chat to find out whether you both have the same ideas about how to look after a baby. (Even though you might privately think you have absolutely no idea about how to care for a baby!) These are the sort of questions you might want to ask:

- Would she want your baby to sleep with her at night (and if so, is this what you want?)?
- Does she have a flexible approach to baby-care (depending on the baby) or is she routine-led?
- Would she like to eat with you and your partner in the evenings and, if so, does she have any special dietary requirements that you will have to cater for?
- Will she do any food shopping if necessary?

Do **not** employ anyone who seems opinionated, talks too much or frightens you! You will be pretty fragile and vulnerable when you come home from hospital and you will find any of the above characteristics stressful. (I've had the most powerful women ringing me from their mobile whilst hiding in the loo, as they have been so intimidated by their maternity nurse.)

Be a little wary of anyone telling you they will 'get' your baby into a routine and sleeping through the night before they leave, especially if you plan to breastfeed. In the early weeks, as far as your baby is concerned, his priorities are to feed (and put on weight) and sleep, rather than to be put on a four-hourly feeding routine. When you find someone you would like to engage, it's a good idea to phone one or two of her recent employers rather than relying only on written references.

A good maternity nurse can give you a really great start – boosting your confidence with your baby, making sure you have a sleep during the day and discreetly ensuring you also have some time with your partner.

Doulas

The aim of a doula is to 'mother the mother' rather than take care of her baby. She has nearly always had children of her own, and is trained to support a woman before, during and after birth. But she is not trained (or 'allowed') to deliver a baby. Many women employ a doula for a few hours a day after they have had their baby – they are a much more flexible option than a maternity nurse, and they will support the mother and her family in any way they can, including cooking and helping with domestic chores. They will also offer advice on feeding and baby-care. At the time of writing, charges are around £20 an hour for qualified doulas. They seem to have become increasingly popular over the last few years, and most women report back that they are incredibly helpful.

Nannies

Employing a nanny is quite a stressful business because she will (hope-fully) live with you for a long time, and become part of your family. Most women employ nannies because they have to go back to work, so their nanny will be in sole charge of their baby. The mother will therefore be understandably anxious that the nanny and the baby get on well. For these reasons, most mothers generally find it better to interview a nanny after, rather than before, their baby has been born – but well before they are due back at work. Then you are able to see how the nanny and your baby respond to each other, and you are back on your feet and in a fit state to make really important decisions.

Focusing on these aspects during pregnancy will not only make things easier for you after the birth on a practical level, but will also get you into the right frame of mind for new motherhood.

CHAPTER 6

thinking ahead about labour

This is an overall view of what's ahead! You might think ignorance is bliss, but it really helps if you consider labour early in pregnancy. It's good to get a general idea of what will go on, and learn how best you can conserve energy and manage it as well as possible. More importantly, if you think about labour in advance, it will also help prepare you for all the different possibilities that might arise – something that is vital if you are going to enjoy it. And you should enjoy it!

For the vast majority of women nature manages the complicated process of birth absolutely perfectly. It is a truly miraculous and totally natural process. But as you will see, especially if it's your first baby, you can't be absolutely sure you are definitely going to have a straightforward birth because it's nothing to do with willpower, how well you have been concentrating on your breathing in your antenatal classes or how much yoga you have done.

For more detail on labour and birth, see Chapters 10–13.

WHAT HAPPENS DURING LABOUR?

The uterus is the shape of a hollow inverted pear – with the wide rounded end pointing upwards and backwards towards the spine, and the narrow bit pointing downwards so it sits at the top of the vagina. The narrow end bit is called the cervix and is an opening that is normally closed. The body of the uterus is made of powerful muscle fibres that can stretch and accommodate a growing baby.

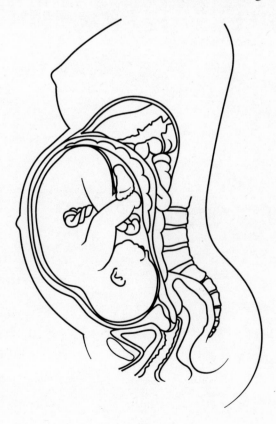

These muscle fibres run longitudinally towards the cervix. It is the cervix that keeps your baby safely in the uterus during pregnancy, so the muscles here are really tough with some circular fibres – a little like a very tight neck of a polo-necked sweater. And within the uterus, think of your baby as though he is lying in fluid (amniotic fluid) contained in a balloon (the membranes).

There are three stages of labour as the uterus has to do three things in order for a baby to be born:

- pull the cervix back over the baby's head and help manoeuvre it into a good position for birth – **First Stage**
- push the baby down the vagina – **Second Stage**
- release and expel the placenta – **Third Stage**

The First Stage of Labour

Two things have to happen:

1 **The muscles of the uterus contract in order to pull back the cervix to widen it and allow the baby's head to pass through to the vagina.**

When labour begins, the muscles of the uterus start rhythmical, regular contractions to flatten (efface) and open (dilate) the cervix. These are labour pains! **Full dilation is 10 cm, the average width of a baby's head.**

For most first-time mothers, the first stage of labour takes fifteen hours (plus or minus six hours). This probably sounds an awfully long time, but nature has a bit of a dilemma. The muscles around the cervix are incredibly tough – they have to be in order to stop the baby, possibly weighing over 9 lb (4 kg) from dropping out before he is ready to be born. This, incidentally, is often the reason why mothers who are expecting twins go into labour early. It's not because twins develop more quickly and are ready to be born earlier than single babies, but because the cervix can't support their double weight.

2 During labour, the contractions of the uterus also have to rotate the baby's head so the top of the back of his head comes first.

During the process of birth, babies, generally speaking, have their chin tucked well down onto their chest, so the top of the back of their head comes first – because this is the narrowest part of the head. The analogy again is the tight polo-necked sweater – if you pull it down over the top of the back of your own head or that of a child, it slips over your head fairly easily; if you put it on over the brow, things are more difficult.

Because of the shape of the female pelvis, at the end of pregnancy babies generally lie looking sideways, facing either of the mother's hips. Broadly speaking, in order to have a trouble-free birth, a baby needs to be lying with his head down and to one side. Yet as the baby moves through the pelvis during labour (chin still on chest) the optimal course is for his head to rotate so that eventually he is born with his face looking downwards. Once the head is delivered, he turns again to look sideways and his body follows this, so the shoulders can be delivered easily. The uterus drives this process. Clever stuff.

This is important information for two reasons. Firstly, gravity is thought to help with the rotation of your baby's head, which is why women are encouraged to stay upright and move around – especially during the early stages of labour. Secondly, although for most babies the business of rotation and birth works perfectly, sometimes babies don't descend into the pelvis in a very good position, which can result in a longer labour or occasionally more serious problems.

One example is that for about 1 in 10 first-time mothers (it is unusual in subsequent labours) their baby 'decides' to move downwards into the pelvis with the back of his head (the occiput) towards her spine rather than orientated towards her hipbone, so when labour starts the uterus has to rotate his head even further before he can be born. This position is called OP – occipito posterior– as opposed to OA – occipito anterior – the normal position. A mother whose baby is lying in an OP position usually (but not always) has a longer and less straightforward labour, and therefore will be more likely to need pain relief than a mother who is carrying a baby in a more usual position.

Occasionally a woman has an awkward-shaped pelvis which isn't very good for childbirth, meaning there isn't enough room for her baby to descend or rotate properly. By the way, don't be fooled by the rather rude expression 'good childbearing hips'. The width of your hips has nothing to do with how roomy your pelvis is. What is relevant is the shape of the bones at the bottom of the pelvis (pelvic outlet) which you and others can't see. From my experience, women who have a 'roomy' pelvis making childbirth quick and easy tend to be of a slight build, tall and apparently narrow-hipped – more the shape of a catwalk model. This is rather irritating for the rest of us.

So – quite simply, the type of labour a woman has is dependent on:

- the shape of her pelvis – over which she has no control
- the position of her baby – over which she has no control

And that's why it's so important to keep an open mind about what sort of birth you would like. If you fall into the 13 per cent of women who need medical help during labour, it won't be your fault!

It is really important to take on board that all of the following descriptions of labour are based on 'Mrs Average' – taking the mean of the labours of a large group of women. So although the next bit is going to be applicable to most of you, it will not be the same for **all** of you! Labours vary enormously from woman to woman and can be most unpredictable, which is why it's sometimes impossible for obstetricians and midwives to foresee how well an individual woman will progress.

The first stage of labour can be subdivided into two sub-stages, according to the degree of dilation of the cervix:

0–3 cm **Latent Stage**
3–10 cm **Active Stage**

Latent Stage

This is the beginning of labour, and during this stage the contractions will flatten (efface) the cervix until it is continuous with the wall of the uterus. When this has happened, you will be around 3 cm dilated. The latent stage is by far the most variable length of time – it's this stage that determines a long or a short labour. The contractions are between 30 and 60 seconds long, and the gap between them varies enormously from woman to woman – from five minutes to twenty minutes apart.

For most women, this early stage of labour will be spent at home and is not too much of a problem as far as pain is concerned – in fact, most mothers report back that it was quite a pleasure. Something is happening at last! The biggest problem for many first-time mothers is that this stage can take a very long time – those girlfriends who tell you that they were in labour for three days but had people for supper (and you think 'Oh my God...') would have had a very long latent stage. Actually, most women have a natural restlessness at this time so having people in for supper is not necessarily as heroic as it sounds. But if you are unlucky enough to spend a whole night not being able to sleep due to mild contractions, followed by a day of more contractions and then yet another night pacing round your sitting room, you will start the active stage very sleep-deprived indeed. In fact, you may need some pain relief just because you are already exhausted.

Conversely, girlfriends who tell you they had an amazingly fast labour of only six hours are likely to have had a 'silent' latent stage – which means they were unaware that the cervix was flattening and dilating. Some women walk around with a cervix dilated at 2 or 3 cm for a week or so before they go straight into active labour. Such is the variability of childbirth.

Active Stage

3–7 cm Dilation

Most women will be in hospital at this stage. From now on, with any luck, the contractions will dilate the cervix at a rate of approximately 1 cm an hour – and this is what your midwife is hoping for. She will give you an internal examination every four hours to check this rate of dilation, and by feeling for the soft spots on your baby's head (fontanelles), she should be able to tell what position your baby is in. You are hoping she will say your baby's head is well flexed, which means his chin is on his chest, as this will help his head pass through the tight polo-neck of the cervix.

At this stage, the contractions become much more powerful and intense. Women will say things like, 'At the beginning, I thought labour was all going to be a piece of cake, and I'd be able to manage perfectly OK with the breathing, but later on the contractions really changed and felt as though they meant serious business.' The contractions lengthen to about 60 seconds and come every three to five minutes. Many women decide that this is the time they would like some pain relief.

7–10 cm Dilation

The contractions become longer still, as the uterus goes into overdrive to pull the cervix back the last couple of centimetres or so. The contractions last between 60 and 90 seconds, and the gap between them closes to every two minutes. But you're nearly there!

Second Stage – Pushing Your Baby Out

This stage lasts round about an hour – and most women have to work hard! The contractions come pretty frequently – every two to four minutes – and last between 60 to 90 seconds. The contractions now have a completely different action – rather than pulling back the cervix, they are pushing your baby down the few inches of the vagina as well as manoeuvring his head into the optimal position for birth.

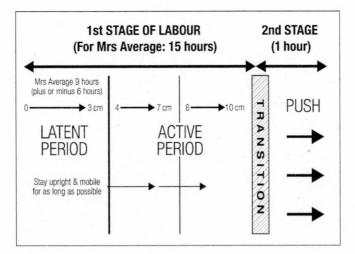

Third Stage – Delivering the Placenta

Once your baby has been born, the uterus will automatically expel the placenta. It takes minutes, rather than hours, and for most women, this bit is an afterthought and hardly worth mentioning…

WHAT CONTRACTIONS REALLY FEEL LIKE

For most women, a contraction starts as a tightening across the tummy and/or lower back. If you have been having Braxton Hicks contractions (see box), labour contractions may start off as more or less the same – the difference being that they become more powerful and don't go away.

Braxton Hicks Contractions

Named after a doctor, hence the odd name, these are mock or practice contractions that every pregnant woman will have, although some women don't notice them. Generally speaking, they are a good thing as they are thought to give the uterus a surge of blood, and this also means a surge of oxygen. Most commonly they feel as though your baby is trying to do a big stretch from inside, and if you put your hand on your tummy, you will feel that it is tight. Or from time to time your tummy may simply feel like a hard ball. Most women will be aware of these practice contractions in the third trimester. This is often when they have been 'overdoing' things or when they lie down, which results in the abdominal muscles relaxing, making the hardening of the uterus more obvious. But if, after reading the above, you still don't think you have ever had one, don't panic that you have a dud uterus – quite a few women tell me that they never experience them. For many women, these 'Braxton Hicks' can become quite intrusive at the end of pregnancy – not exactly painful, but strong enough for you to stop what you are doing.

So for some women, early labour contractions may be just an extension of Braxton Hicks contractions. As labour progresses, the contractions for most women have a definite pattern – during each one the hardening around the tummy becomes stronger and stronger, reaches a peak and then starts to unwind or abate…until it has disappeared completely (see the diagram opposite). As labour progresses, the contractions last longer and become progressively powerful, with the gap between them becoming shorter. In my antenatal classes, I always ask second-time mothers to describe what their contractions felt like when they were having their first baby. They don't say, 'I wasn't expecting them to feel like that!' but women do say, 'I was completely unprepared for the intensity of the contractions. The tightening seemed to take over my whole body!' At the end of labour, many women describe a contraction as though their tummy is encased in two steel bands, like a vice with a rotating clamp each side, and the bands are gradually being tightened. The pain is not only felt in the tummy area but can radiate over to your back. And at the peak, it can feel a little like being on a theme park roller coaster – your body is completely taken over. **But when the contraction has passed, you are completely back to your normal self.**

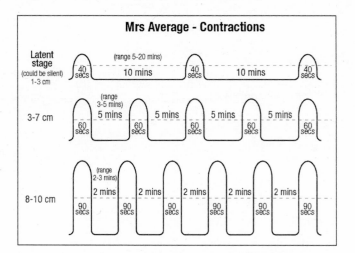

BREATHING AND 'RELAXATION' DURING LABOUR

The longitudinal muscles of the uterus contract in order to flatten (efface) the cervix and then pull it back over your baby's head. When a muscle in your body contracts involuntarily (like cramp) it is painful, so contractions during labour are painful for most women. However, it is important to remember it's the pain of something going right rather than the pain of something going wrong!

When you are in pain, you do two things instinctively:

- hold your breath
- tighten all your muscles

Cast your mind back to very old films showing women in labour. The woman lies flat on her back on a large brass bed. As she has a contraction, she hangs onto the rails at the top end, tightens all her muscles, screams and then holds her breath. She can't hold her breath for more than a minute or so, but the contraction hasn't yet passed, so she ends it with panting and more anguished sounds. If you did all this for 15 hours when NOT in labour you would be exhausted...but if you do this as well as being in labour you are going to be doubly exhausted and not exactly at your best when the time comes to push out your baby.

So as soon as a contraction starts you are going to do two things to counteract these instinctive responses:

- keep breathing (as opposed to breath-holding)
- keep all your muscles as relaxed as possible, so the uterus can get on with its work

Basic Breathing in Labour

This is very simple:

- Breathe in through your nose and out through your mouth.
- Fix your eyes on something (perhaps the second hand of a clock if you're timing the contractions) and breathe directly 'at' it.
- Keep your breathing as slow as possible and try and breathe in the same amount that you breathe out.

- At the end of the contraction, say goodbye to it by giving an audible sigh. This will keep your oxygen and carbon dioxide levels balanced, so you don't over-breathe (hyperventilate) and feel dizzy.

I asked Lorin, who obviously delivers babies every day, to write about 'labour generally' from an obstetrician's point of view.

LABOUR AND DELIVERY – THE MEDICAL PERSPECTIVE
(by Lorin Lakasing)

The three most important pieces of advice I would give anyone to help them get the best out of their labour and to make it a truly memorable event for all the right reasons are as follows:

1. Keep an Open Mind

Clearly it is reasonable to have some idea of how you want your labour to go, and many women write a birth plan to help guide the professionals looking after them. However, labour is a very dynamic process and things can change quickly so you too must be willing to change your plan accordingly and accept professional advice. Remember, this may be your first labour but it is probably the 10th baby your midwife has delivered this week. She has seen it all before, so trust her judgement. Believe me – she is on your side. Being too didactic about what you want and don't want can result in a large mismatch between expectation and reality, which inevitably leads to disappointment and frustration for all concerned. Worse still, if you have very strong views this can adversely affect your outcome, and after all what everyone wants is a safe delivery and a happy and healthy (albeit exhausted!) mother and a well baby.

CHRISTINE HILL'S PREGNANCY GUIDE

2. Do not Compare Your Birthing Experience with those of Others

This is an almost inevitable mistake for all first-time mothers. After all, you've never done this before so why shouldn't you listen to your mother or sister or neighbour? Well don't, because for all that they mean well, they are giving advice from a subjective perspective based on a small number of personal experiences. If you have concerns or worries, talk to the professionals who do this day in and day out. The information you will get is much more accurate and a lot less scary. Just because your neighbour delivered a 9 lb baby last month with no pain relief, it does not mean you should feel a failure for requesting an epidural. There might be all sorts of reasons why your labour is more prolonged and difficult, such as the position of the baby's head as he engages in the birth canal.

3. Get Clued up in Advance

If you want to know about the pros and cons of having an epidural, for example, the time to ask is not when you are in the throes of advanced labour. You won't be taking in the answers and you certainly won't appreciate the delay in getting you comfortable whilst the anaesthetist chats to you about these matters!

Similarly, the point at which the obstetrician comes into your room and decides that delivery by Caesarean section is required is not the first time to have thought about this. It is perfectly possible to have had a brief discussion with your midwife about these things, even if you are at very low risk, just so you are prepared. Women who have taken the trouble to do this are much more likely to feel that they are in the driving seat and part of the decision making. Think of it as the aeroplane emergency drill prior to takeoff!

Sometimes you might need medical intervention...

Induction of Labour

This is when your labour is stimulated with medicines so that delivery is expedited sooner than it would be without intervention. There are very clear medical indications for obstetricians to recommend this to some women. Women usually have two main concerns about induction: firstly, the level of intervention this procedure results in, and secondly, the increased likelihood of delivery by Caesarean section. Induction of labour is inevitably associated with a longer stay in hospital, more monitoring and more vaginal examinations. So there is no getting away from the increased rate of intervention. But very often, the reason why induction has been recommended to you is in itself a reason to be monitored in hospital, so it is just a matter of accepting that this is part of the deal. What matters is that both you and your baby are well at the end of the day. And as for the likelihood of delivery by Caesarean section, it really does depend on why and at what gestation you are being induced, and your obstetrician will be able to give you more personalised advice about this. So try not to be negative about induction of labour and remember that it has been recommended to you because the benefits outweigh the risks (see page 170).

Caesarean Section

Much has been written in the press about the rising rate of Caesarean section, not only in the UK but throughout the developed world too. In some maternity units where predominantly high-risk pregnancies are cared for, the Caesarean section rate is over 20 per cent, and these women with complicated pregnancies have accepted early on in the antenatal period that this is the safest method of delivery for them. However, for the low-risk woman who has avoided any medical input so far and is labouring away at term, to be unexpectedly faced with the prospect of delivery by Caesarean section can be both alarming and disappointing.

Caesarean section can be performed for a number of reasons.

Emergency Caesarean: The Decision is Taken When You are in Labour

Sometimes there is no rush in expediting delivery – for example, when you are not progressing in labour despite every effort (usually this is because the baby's head is stuck in the wrong position), and in these situations you are transferred to the operating theatre calmly and you have more time to get your head around the events or to ask any questions. Sometimes the situation is a bit more dramatic – for instance, there are signs that the baby is getting distressed or you may be bleeding, and clearly in these situations there is less chat and more immediate action. This can be quite scary for both you and your partner, but the best thing you can do is try to remain calm and remember that whilst you may be feeling out of control, the people who are looking after you do this every day of their lives.

Also, try not to be put out by the number of people in the theatre. There are at least seven people involved in a Caesarean section: the obstetrician (who performs the procedure), the surgical assistant (who helps the obstetrician), the anaesthetist (who makes sure you are pain-free for the procedure), the anaesthetic nurse (who helps the anaesthetist), the scrub nurse (who hands the instruments and swabs to the obstetrician), the midwife (who receives the baby) and the paediatrician (who checks baby at delivery). Everyone in the operating theatre (including your partner!) will be dressed in surgical blues. This scene may be a far cry from the dim lighting of your cosy delivery room with just your partner and midwife present, but if you take time to imagine it before you go into labour, in the unlikely event that you end up there, you might surprise yourself and others as to how calm and confident you can be (see page 211).

Elective Caesarean: The Decision is Taken During Pregnancy, Rather Than When you are in Labour

This is pretty straightforward – the following problems are reasons for an elective Caesarean, because a vaginal birth is simply a non-viable or dangerous option:

- your baby is in a transverse position (lying with his head and bottom facing each of your hips) making birth impossible
- your baby is breech – see page 166
- placenta praevia – the placenta is in front of your baby's head, making birth dangerous (page 50)
- twins, with one baby breech or transverse – or just to be on the safe side
- triplets – when goodness knows what may happen to the position of the second and third baby
- various medical conditions that the mother may have

Alternatively, you may have decided that is the best option for you (see page 30).

You will usually be booked in for a Caesarean a week or so before your due date – simply because it is much safer for staff to operate on a non-contracting uterus, and at a time when everyone is calm and prepared, rather than as an emergency.

Premature Delivery

Overall, about 7 per cent of babies are born prematurely. This figure is much higher in maternity units where there are intensive care facilities for newborns on site. If you have developed complications in the antenatal period and your obstetrician anticipates early delivery, your care will be transferred to such a unit. In this situation there will be plenty of time to discuss and plan this. However, if you unexpectedly go into labour at a very early gestation, you may need to be transferred promptly, often in an ambulance, to an appropriate unit where your baby can be cared for safely. Every attempt is made to transfer you to a unit that is as near to your home and family as possible, although intensive care cots are in short supply, and many units in the UK are closing down in order to centralise resources. Just remember that you are being transferred in the interests of your baby as it is much safer to transfer whilst the baby is still inside you than to move a vulnerable newborn who is just a few hours old.

Depending on how premature your baby is and the cause of your preterm labour, both you and baby may need close medical surveillance and care before and after delivery. You will usually be reviewed by a neonatologist (a paediatrician who specialises in the care of unwell newborns) in anticipation of a premature delivery, and this doctor will tell you what you can expect and what investigations and treatments might be carried out on baby after delivery. Your obstetrician will decide the most appropriate time and way to deliver your baby. Premature delivery is very stressful for parents as it calls upon your patience, and forces you to deal with uncertainty. As ever, good communication and consistent advice from professionals is important. And remember, just because you have delivered prematurely and your care has been largely medical, it is still important for your midwife to be involved as you will need ongoing care when you get home. In particular, you will need help and support with breastfeeding, which is arguably more important for premature babies than those born at term.

As well as thinking ahead about labour, don't forget to think about life after the birth and bringing your baby home. While it is important to be prepared for what might happen during the birth, focusing on the days and weeks with your new baby will help keep everything in perspective.

CHAPTER 7

well-meant advice (and dire warnings)

You will have noticed that you are the target for a great deal of advice about what and, particularly, what not to do when you are pregnant. Quite a bit of this is couched in finger-wagging terms and a great deal is unnecessarily alarming. Society now regards the pregnant woman as its collective property and also seems to relish treating pregnant women as foolish children who need to clean up their act, or else... There are dire warnings about the risks of this and that, and many women I see are seriously anxious about whether they have already caused their baby grievous bodily harm in a casual moment.

Official bodies give advice about what you should or shouldn't eat or drink when you are pregnant. They play very safe indeed! Usually the issue is that a food or drink or smoking represents a risk to the fetus or the pregnancy – but what is often not said is how big a risk exists, especially if it is indulged in only occasionally. And some women and some pregnancies are more vulnerable than others. Studies disagree with each other, varying from country to country and year to year as to, for instance, what level of alcohol intake is 'safe'. It's all really difficult to unpick. Advice from official bodies is not tailored to you as an individual; it's meant to cover absolutely everybody. Unfortunately, it tends to come across as rules that must not be broken, rather than well-meant advice enabling you to use informed discretion.

Not only do mothers start to worry about what they have done in error, more insidiously they can also come to believe that if they avoid all the risks and hazards in what they eat or what they do, it will ensure they have a perfect pregnancy and baby. It just can't. Sadly, no-one knows the causes of most stillbirths, for instance. Whatever you do, you simply can't guarantee that all the things that can possibly go wrong during pregnancy will never happen. You just have to remind yourself that they usually don't, especially after 14 weeks. Nothing you do will definitely produce a perfect pregnancy, but most pregnancies and most babies are fine.

Obviously, you want to do the best for your baby and avoid putting him at risk. But if you unintentionally eat something on a 'must avoid' list, stay calm! Most advice about what to avoid is over-cautious because it prohibits rather than advising you on the size of any risk, which is usually very small.

Nevertheless, there are uncommon, though real, risks to the pregnancy and fetus which can be limited and are to do with what you take into your body. They fall into two main groups: food-borne infections and toxins.

FOOD-BORNE INFECTIONS

Some infections, contracted by eating contaminated food, are potentially hazardous to your pregnancy. Sometimes they cause miscarriage or premature labour, or they may cross the placenta and infect your baby.

The risk of getting a potentially dangerous infection from food is a lottery. There is always a small chance of the relevant contaminating germ being in soft unpasteurised cheese, unwashed salad or whatever, so completely cutting these out makes sense, as you can otherwise never be sure it isn't there in any portion. This is different from the issue with toxins (caffeine, mercury, alcohol and so on, see below) where the risk increases with how much you take in. Complete avoidance of foods in which there is a definite risk is actually good advice, though at the same time such infections are rare, so a slip-up is unlikely to be disastrous.

The sheer volume of advice on what not to eat or cook is breathtaking – and at the very least you could be in for an orgy of hand-washing. But there are alarming inconsistencies between the lists – probably because each includes foods for which there is only weak evidence for avoidance as well as other foods for which the evidence is strong. You (and your husband) can fall into the trap of adding all the lists together and allowing apprehension to spoil every meal you have. I have spent literally days (together with my husband who is a university professor and medical academic) trying to make sense of all the advice on what is inevitably dangerous if eaten when pregnant (nothing is – apart from arsenic, cyanide or weedkiller and so on) and what is 'sensible' advice (the 'safest' advice might be not to eat at all).

In my opinion, arrived at after a great deal of discussion and research, you can pretty well eat your normal balanced diet with only a very few exceptions and simple precautions. And if you have actually eaten one of the exceptions ('You mean you forgot to wash the pre-packed salad!'; 'We didn't ask the waiter if the chicken was properly cooked') don't panic; the chances of getting an infection are minuscule.

There are two main infections that can cause trouble – listeriosis and toxoplasmosis. You may also read about salmonella (and be advised not to eat raw eggs and so on, see below) but the hard evidence for this being a significant risk for your pregnancy is not convincing.

Listeriosis

Listeriosis is caused by listeria bacteria, which are occasionally present in certain foods but are **killed by proper cooking or full pasteurisation**. It is a rare disease, presenting as a mild flu-like illness, sometimes with diarrhoea. During pregnancy it can, but doesn't always, infect not only the mother but her baby as well, and cause miscarriage, premature delivery or stillbirth. If diagnosed, it can be safely treated by intravenous antibiotics in hospital.

Obviously, you will want to take reasonable steps to avoid listeria infection – but let's look at exactly how likely this is. In 2006 there were 722,500 births in the UK but only 25 cases of pregnant women who contracted listeriosis. That fits with the usually cited risk of about 1 in 20–30,000 pregnancies. You can see that the risk is really, really tiny. Nevertheless, to avoid possibly contaminated food, you should try to make sure any cooked food you eat is **cooked adequately** and try not to eat the following:

- unpasteurised cheese – it will say so on the label
- blue-veined cheese (such as Dolcelatte, Danish blue, Stilton)
- soft cheeses with skins
- pâté

Here, I know, I am falling into the trap of giving the safest possible advice – not to eat this or that even when the risk is tiny. But the list is short, based on bacteriological evidence, consistency and logic – and it's reasonably easy to live for nine months without unpasteurised cheese. Yet if, in a pregnancy moment, you unintentionally eat any of the above or are unsure whether you had heated something up adequately, *do not panic* because the chances are overwhelmingly great that nothing will happen to you or your baby. But if you develop a temperature or feel really fluey in the following few days call your GP.

All in all? Stick to hard cheese without blue bits and don't eat pâté.

Toxoplasmosis

This is even rarer than listeriosis in pregnancy itself (about 1 in 50,000 pregnancies) though nearly half of the UK population will have toxoplasmosis at some time in their lives. Most people don't know that they have had it so you might well have had it before you became pregnant and are now immune. When it happens it is a simple, brief, flu-like illness. If a woman is pregnant and catches it for the first time there is about a 40 per cent chance that her fetus will be infected, which may result in miscarriage or damage to the developing eyes and nervous system.

Toxoplasmosis is caused by an organism found mainly in cat

faeces or the meat and bodily fluids from infected lambs, cows and goats. This includes their urine or excrement on vegetables. Cooking kills it. Here is some more 'safest possible' advice, which is actually easy to follow.

Avoid eating:

- raw or very rare (pink) meat (wash your hands after handling raw meat)
- unwashed salads and vegetables
- goats' milk (not too difficult to avoid)

And:

- Wash your hands well if you unintentionally handle cats' poo, and wear gloves if you are gardening where cats might defecate.
- Don't go near sheep or lambs at lambing time (not too difficult for most, though not all, of us…)

All in all? No pink meat and wash your hands, salad and veg a lot.

Other Warnings

Raw Eggs?

There is a minuscule risk of contracting salmonella from imported raw eggs, such as may be used in home-made mayonnaise or mousse. But eggs with a 'lion' mark are almost certainly salmonella-free. There have been fewer than 20 cases reported in the international scientific literature of a pregnant woman contracting salmonella and miscarrying. This is very rare indeed. But it might be worth avoiding fresh mayonnaise and mousse if you are on holiday abroad.

Coleslaw?

As coleslaw contains raw cabbage, you would want to ensure the cabbage had been well washed before preparation, just in case an infected goat may have peed on it. It also just might contain raw imported egg if the mayonnaise was home-made. Neither seems to me to be a major risk but it would seem a sensible precaution to buy your coleslaw from a reliable source, such as an upmarket supermarket rather than a dubious deli.

Seafood?

Seafood, including cooked shellfish, is good for developing babies but raw shellfish can give you food poisoning from time to time, as everyone knows. It is often said that food poisoning is particularly unpleasant when you are pregnant but I can't find good evidence that it is a risk to your baby. It is OK to eat sushi.

TOXINS

The issue here is one of degree. There is no point in panicking about accidental minimal exposure ('Oh my God, I've just bitten into a liqueur chocolate...' or 'Terrible news – someone is smoking a cigarette in the corner of this room'). This is a quite different issue from the small lottery chance of eating something that might be contaminated and infect you. Here the key problem is how much toxin is risky for you and your baby.

Smoking

Numerous studies show that smoking is not only a risk to you but also to your baby and his placenta. Smoking in pregnancy increases the risk of miscarriage, poor growth, stillbirth, cot death, respiratory problems and even death in infancy and so on. Not surprisingly, official advice is not to smoke at all.

Although the risk from the occasional cigarette is something that is not known, it seems sensible to recommend that if you still haven't given up, now is definitely the best time to do so, and if your partner smokes, it will be easiest if you give up together.

Alcohol

This is quite a difficult one to disentangle. We know, for instance, that alcohol is a definite toxin as far as the developing fetus is concerned. And then there is the finding that different levels of alcohol present different risks to the baby, and these change according to how far the pregnancy has developed. The amount of regular alcohol required to increase the rate of miscarriage is an awful lot smaller than that needed to increase the risk of fetal alcohol syndrome (see below). Excessive and regular alcohol drinking in the first trimester increases the risk of miscarriage but doesn't seem to do so in the second and third trimesters. The risk of miscarriage in the first trimester (but not later) is probably increased at a regular intake of two units a day but different studies suggest different levels. Below two units a day, the risks to pregnancy and baby are unclear.

The Department of Health and the British Medical Association both recommend that women who are pregnant (or indeed trying to conceive!) should not drink any alcohol at all. But the Royal

College of Obstetricians and Gynaecologists and the Food Standards Agency advise that there is no evidence of harm from low levels of alcohol consumption – defined as no more than one or two units once or twice a week. Draft guidance from NICE (National Institute for Health and Clinical Excellence) indicates that the threshold for alcohol consumption once or twice a week is: half a pint of ordinary strength beer or cider, one small glass of wine (smaller than a glass you would pour yourself), one alcopop or a pub measure of spirits.

Alcohol that crosses the placenta in large quantities regularly will increase the risk of (though not inevitably cause) miscarriage, still-birth, poor fetal growth, premature birth, congenital abnormalities and psychological problems in the baby. Notoriously, it can cause a condition called fetal alcohol syndrome. The babies and then children with this syndrome have abnormal facial features, growth deficiency, small heads and intellectual impairment – for which there is no cure. The number of children who have this syndrome is tiny – 100–150 cases each year are recorded in England. However, the risk of this condition is related to drinking more than six units every day during pregnancy – which I would have thought is going for it.

Obviously, the prevention rate for conditions related to alcohol consumed during pregnancy would be 100 per cent if pregnant women drank no alcohol at all. In the same vein, there would be hardly any skin cancer if no-one was allowed out of the house when the sun was shining. One question is whether this means that the occasional lapse, or drinking at a party when you were just pregnant and did not know it, means your baby is damaged. The answer to that is almost certainly no.

Many women go right off alcohol when they are pregnant in any case. They may be the lucky ones. But if this doesn't happen to you, there is no hard evidence that the occasional glass of wine will harm your baby. The choice has to be yours.

And Cocaine, Crack, Cannabis and Other Illegals?

Don't do it – although there is poor evidence of any danger from moderate use, it isn't worth the risk since these substances will have a direct impact on the fetal brain.

Mercury

There are high levels of mercury in fish at the top of the marine food chain so avoid shark, marlin or swordfish – not too difficult. Tuna is OK in moderation – it's difficult to be precise about a threshold, but once a week would appear to be safe.

Caffeine

Found, of course, in coffee, tea, some fizzy drinks and chocolate. The main risk associated with a high intake of caffeine is miscarriage in the first trimester, but different studies have identified wildly varying levels of caffeine that might present a risk. While writing this chapter, for instance, two new studies have been reported – one showing no risk of miscarriage from moderate caffeine intake, the other suggesting an increased rate of miscarriage among women drinking more than a small cup of coffee a day. With such disparate results it seems more reasonable to opt for a middle path than prohibit coffee altogether. The Food Standards Agency currently suggests a daily limit of 300 mg: this means your day can, for instance, contain one coffee (100 mg), three teas (50 mg each) and either a coke or a chocolate bar (50 mg each).

Too Much Vitamin A – and Liver

You, and your baby, need vitamin A for adequate sight and growth, and a normal healthy diet provides this. But too much is bad news for your baby (though an exceptionally rare problem), and there are studies linking a (very) high intake of vitamin supplements while pregnant with a small increase in the rate of abnormalities in the baby. With this in mind, don't take cod liver oil or non-pregnancy vitamin supplements.

Warnings: a Summary

Wash

- Veg, salad and fruit grown near the ground
- Your hands after handling raw meat
- Your hands after touching cat poo

Don't eat

- Raw or pink meat
- Unpasteurised, soft or blue-veined cheese
- Pâté

Maximum daily intake (probably halve quantities in first trimester)

- Half a glass of wine
- Three cups of coffee or six cups of tea (fewer if mugs)

Don't

- Smoke
- Garden in bare hands
- Take non-pregnancy vitamin supplements

And: keep away from lambs, goats' milk and eating big fierce fish.

It is often said that you shouldn't eat liver, especially calves' liver, because this contains a high quantity of vitamin A. Chicken liver contains about half as much. Official health bodies recommend abstinence during pregnancy, though food scientists are much less consistent, pointing out that there is no clear evidence that a high liver consumption (as opposed to too many vitamin supplements) is unsafe. I suppose it would seem sensible (although cautious) not to buy liver for supper or order liver in a restaurant, though not to worry if you eat some unintentionally.

WHAT YOU SHOULD EAT

The simplest thing to say is 'stick to your normal balanced diet'. The Food Standards Agency and the Department of Health *Pregnancy Book* give sensible advice if you are feeling uncertain about this, but to me it doesn't seem to need any more than common sense.

You should take a folic acid supplement for the first three months, and some, mainly dark-skinned, women will be advised to take a vitamin D supplement. If you eat a healthy diet you don't need vitamin supplements but if you can't resist the temptation, only take those suitable for pregnancy.

There is disagreement about whether you should take any omega-3 supplements. Almost certainly this is because it depends on how much omega-3 you obtain from your normal diet. If you eat oily fish (salmon, mackerel, sardines) twice a week then you don't need them. Don't take cod liver oil.

Safety Issues in Essential Body Maintenance

It is OK (thank goodness) to:

- get your highlights done

- have a facial

- wax your legs and bikini line

- have laser hair removal

- have a manicure and pedicure

- use face creams bought over the counter

- use fake tan

In the UK it is sometimes advised that you avoid Jacuzzis, saunas or steam rooms during the first trimester. Although there isn't a good body of hard evidence to justify this, there is a theoretical risk of miscarriage if an early pregnancy is exposed to a high temperature.

There are so many scare stories about the dangers for the unborn child from diet, drugs, infections and so on that it is very difficult to imagine how women ever managed to have a healthy baby before all this advice was available. It might be worth remembering that your grandmothers didn't have any of the above guidance!

CHAPTER 8

muscles and bones

Your front, back and undercarriage are vital muscles that need to be looked after! There are two groups of muscles that quite literally take most of the strain during pregnancy – the pelvic floor muscles and the abdominals (tummy muscles). It's worth giving specific attention to these during pregnancy because of their importance to you afterwards – they will be with you long after your baby has grown up and left home.

PELVIC FLOOR MUSCLES

Because I'm a physiotherapist who has specialised in women's health (and therefore problems), I have to start off with these muscles. Women are absolutely dependent on them!

The pelvis contains and protects organs such as the bladder, uterus and lower bowel. The floor of the pelvis is the area between your legs and is formed by an arrangement of several muscles, known as the pelvic floor, which support these organs. The muscles also allow three openings to pass through – the anus, the vagina and the urethra (through which you pee).

If these muscles weaken and sag, they can no longer support the contents of the pelvis and will not help the openings close off properly, causing embarrassing problems. The most common of these is stress incontinence – inadvertently wetting yourself when coughing, sneezing or laughing. The more serious complications include prolapse, which is when the uterus starts to sag down into the vagina, or the vaginal walls collapse under pressure from a full bladder or bowel.

The whole business of having a baby puts the pelvic floor muscles under enormous strain. They have to cope with the increasing weight of a pregnant uterus and then a huge amount of stretching to allow the baby through the vaginal opening. Most women will have bruised and sore pelvic floor muscles after giving birth, and many will find that they have stitches. You will need to do pelvic floor exercises (also called Kegel exercises) as soon as possible after your baby has been born in order to help the muscles recover – even following a Caesarean birth. Exercising your pelvic floor plays a vital part in accelerating the healing process and getting your muscles back to their pre-pregnancy state (or even better).

If you get into the habit of doing pelvic floor exercises whilst you are pregnant, you will be familiar with the routine and won't have to learn how to do a new exercise immediately after birth when the muscles will be sore. It is a good idea to try and 'programme' yourself during pregnancy to contract your pelvic floor muscles every day. If you are familiar with contracting and relaxing these muscles, you will also be able to relax them more effectively when your baby is being born, which will help his delivery.

How to Do a Pelvic Floor Contraction

Squeeze and lift the following:

- the anal sphincter muscles – as though you need to stop a potential fart
- the opening of the vagina – as though you are trying to stop a tampon falling out
- the urethra area – imagining you have a full bladder but the loo is engaged

Think of the above as a unit and hold the contraction of the whole unit for a slow count of two. Then relax the muscles, and you should feel a slight 'drop' between your legs as the muscles return to their former position. If you can feel this drop, then you have successfully contracted your pelvic floor muscles. Neither your buttock muscles nor your eyebrows should be working at the same time! The above is a basic pelvic floor contraction – which will keep the muscles toned.

During pregnancy, contract and relax your pelvic floor in groups of five contractions at a time, at least five times a day. This will make a total of 25 contractions a day. Don't worry about trying to hold the contractions (so called 'sustained contractions') if you find it difficult – your pelvic floor has enough to cope with trying to support the weight of your baby so holding for a count of two seconds is enough at this stage. I would leave the sustained contractions until after you have had your baby and need to rehabilitate the muscles (for more on this, see my book *A Perfect Start*, published by Vermilion).

When to Do Pelvic Floor Exercises

- standing in a queue
- waiting for websites to download
- stuck at red traffic lights
- listening to someone very boring at a party
- waiting on the phone: 'Your call is very important to us...'

Hopefully, none of the above is news to you. You may already be an old hand at pelvic floor exercises or will have started them during yoga or other classes. It doesn't take a genius to realise that these muscles also play a major role in your sex life.

Wise women will continue to do 10 lifts a day for the rest of their lives as a 'well-woman' exercise to keep the muscles in good working order. Toned pelvic floor muscles are the best insurance against future problems – when your 'baby' goes off to university, you will still have the same set of muscles – and no woman in her 60s, let alone 50s expects to wear a pad because she leaks wee when she coughs or laughs.

ABDOMINAL MUSCLES

Your back and your front are connected! Contrary to what you might think, tummy muscles actually protect your lower back, and if you have weak abdominal muscles you will almost certainly get backache. This is because they are anchored to and help stabilise the back of your ribcage, pelvis and spine.

Your abdominals are in three layers. The two deep layers are like a large corset or tube – attached to the bottom of most of the ribcage, spine and pelvis. On top of these layers are two strap muscles (called recti: nothing to do with rectum!), which run vertically down the front of your tummy from the breastbone to your pubic bone (symphysis pubis). Abdominal muscles are designed not only to give you a flat tummy, but by acting with the buttock muscles, they also line up the angle of the pelvis correctly with the lower spine to protect the spine from too much 'hollowing'.

Now this clearly is a problem for most pregnant women – their abdominals will have to stretch over the bump of the growing baby. This makes it difficult for the abdominals and the back muscles to keep in balance. Because the stretched abdominals are too stretched to hold the pelvis consistently in the correct position, it usually tilts forwards, like a bucket, resulting in the normal hollowing in the small of your back becoming more pronounced. This in turn results in low backache, especially at the end of pregnancy.

How to Prevent Low Backache

Firstly, take off your clothes and stand sideways in front of a long mirror, so you can see the whole of your back from the side. Let your tummy slob out and see how the hollowing in your lower back increases. Then pull your lower tummy muscles in as tight as possible, and you will see that they pull up the front of the pelvis (as in the diagram overleaf) and flatten the hollowing. Your posture is now better, your back is protected and at the same time you are doing your best to keep the tone in your stretched abdominals. If you have trouble with this, try the following:

Stand with your back against a wall and the heels of your feet an inch or two away from the skirting. Pull your tummy muscles in so that the small of your back touches the wall. You will feel a pull in your lower tummy muscles, which is the movement you want to do.

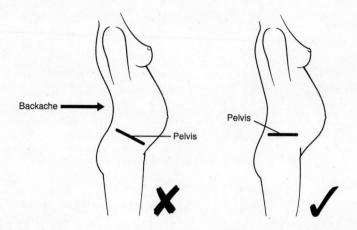

So the message is: when you are standing and walking, pull in your tummy muscles and **try and make yourself look two months less pregnant than you are**. Think of this as 'cuddling' your baby with your tummy muscles – you won't squash or harm him! Getting into this habit is better than trying to do active abdominal strengthening exercises – good posture and good muscle tone are more important than muscle power during pregnancy.

Incidentally, buying an over-the-counter elastic pregnancy belt isn't the brilliant solution it might seem! A belt will support your tummy muscles, but will also do their work – so when you are wearing one, your muscles don't have to work at all and will become weaker. On the whole, it's better not to wear one unless a physiotherapist has suggested it.

Looking after Your Strap Muscles (Recti)

Under normal circumstances, when you do a sit-up your abdominals – particularly the two strap muscles – contract. But as soon as your baby is big enough to make a visible bulge when you are lying on your back, your strap muscles are compromised by having to stretch over the bump, and they lose their leverage. What happens is that they try and do the work of pulling you upright, but at a certain point the bulk of the baby makes them bulge outwards or 'peak' in the middle. Finally, a different muscle group (the hip flexors to be precise) takes over. Meanwhile, the poor old strap muscles have had more strain put on them, and are in danger of becoming over-stretched and losing some of their elasticity. You might notice this happen when you try to sit up in the bath. There is also a thin sheet of tissue down the middle of your tummy, helping to keep the two strap muscles together. If the muscles are overstretched, this tissue will also become stretched and very thin, making it difficult to regain a flat tummy after your baby's birth. Although this is not a disaster and sometimes cannot be helped (especially if you are of short build yourself, carrying a big baby or expecting twins), it seems sensible to take steps to try and prevent it happening by avoiding certain sitting-up movements.

So, in order to protect these strap muscles, **avoid doing any sit-ups once your pregnancy shows**. This means:

- rolling over to one side before getting out of bed (in the middle of the night for yet another pee) and letting your arms rather than your tummy muscles push you upright
- when you need to sit up in the bath, use a grab rail – they are unfashionable at the moment, but very useful when you are

pregnant. If things become hopelessly difficult, it may be possible to attach a rope to the taps to haul yourself up with. Obviously, you can take a shower instead, but at the end of pregnancy most women will say that a shower is not quite the same thing as a bath...

Lifting

Some of you will be told you mustn't lift anything heavy when you are pregnant as it might cause a miscarriage. This is an old wives' tale – you won't miscarry, but you do need to take care and lift correctly as your lower back is particularly vulnerable now you are pregnant (see above).

Actually, if you get into the habit of always lifting properly now, this will stand you in good stead for the rest of your life. When you lift something (even if it's not at all heavy) always go down on one knee, and when you stand up, pull in your tummy muscles and **keep your back straight**. In theory you can of course squat – but this is not always practical when you are heavily pregnant or wearing a tight

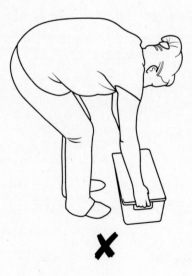

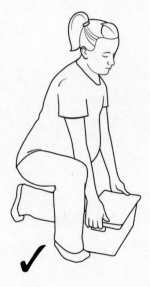

skirt. Keeping your back straight applies to getting something from a low cupboard, whether at work or in your kitchen. It also applies to loading or unpacking a washing machine and dishwasher, something you probably do every day.

Dishwashers are always put on the floor rather than on top of something. Loading and unloading them makes you bend down and straighten up in a way that puts a strain on your back. Considering that 80 per cent of women suffer from backache at some time, I wonder if dishwashers are still on the floor because kitchens are designed by men or by women who haven't had children. It isn't possible to unpack a dishwasher while you are on one knee, as there is nowhere to put the clean stuff – but it is perfectly possible to mount a dishwasher on a low cupboard, so the bottom shelf is at waist height when the door is open. And a microwave then fits perfectly on the top. If you are ever in the position to redesign your kitchen, I suggest you do the same. I have had several letters from women who came to me many years ago and wanted to let me know that they have raised their dishwasher and it has changed their life.

Meanwhile, ask your husband to do dishwasher duties whilst you are pregnant and for the first few months after you have had the baby. And, perhaps, thereafter.

High Heels

Although these might be vital for your self-esteem, they are not going to help prevent you getting backache. In order to stay upright when wearing heels, you have to lean backwards a little bit – so when you are pregnant, the hollowing in your lower back becomes even more accentuated. If you look at your posture in a long mirror with and without high heels, you will see what I mean. So it's best to try and get used to wearing flattish or at least flatter shoes during pregnancy. But if you don't feel properly dressed without heels, they probably won't do much harm for the occasional hour or so.

Sitting

A good chair should support your lower back and your whole foot should rest comfortably on the floor. Shoving a bulky pillow between your lower back and the chair is not necessarily the answer, as doing this can make the hollow in your back rather worse. You should sit fairly upright, rather than 'slouch', so your body weight is taken through your pelvis, rather than through your tail bone right at the base of your spine (coccyx).

A few women experience a very painful tail bone, and it hurts when sitting down or getting up from sitting. This is called coccydynia (or coccygodynia) – and it can be the result of an old injury,

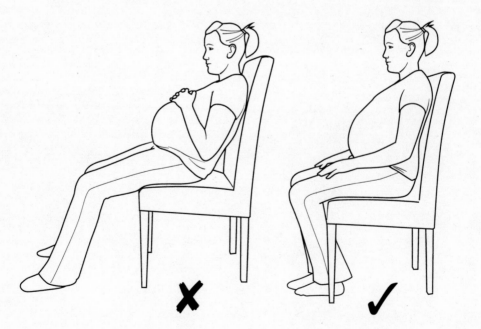

or spontaneously occur at the end of pregnancy. If you bruised or fractured your coccyx before becoming pregnant, it's important that this information is recorded in your notes before delivery, because birth will put a strain on it. During pregnancy there isn't much that can be done – like most things it should get better after your baby has been born. Just at the moment you will need to sit on a well-padded seat (or sit on a pillow if you can find one that helps) and avoid sitting for too long. Your sitting position is especially important if you are at a computer for long periods.

First Aid for Low Backache

If your back is aching at the end of the day, try the following exercise, which is called a pelvic tilt:

- Lie on your back on your bed or on the floor, with your head on a pillow and your knees bent.
- Tighten your tummy muscles to flatten the small of your back against the floor or mattress.
- Relax the muscles then repeat twice.

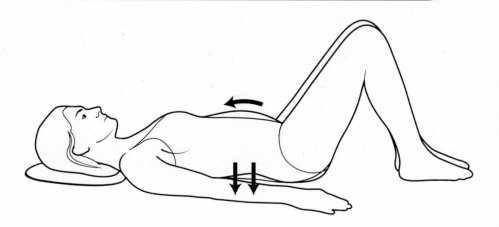

High Backache

As your baby grows, the lower ribs have to move outwards and upwards to allow him more room. Many women find their whole ribcage gets bigger – and their bras, shirts and jackets become too tight. The ribs are all attached to the upper spine by means of a system of tiny joints. The displacement of the ribs can result in pain in these joints – typically to one side of the spine at the level of the bottom of your shoulder blade.

Sometimes, just going for a swim will mobilise the joint and relieve the pain. Otherwise, try the following exercise:

- Sit on a chair. Bend your elbows and put the palms of your hands to rest on your ribcage above your breasts. Lift your elbows so they are in a straight line with your shoulders (see picture below).
- Bend your spine sideways – twice to one side and then twice to the other side.
- Turn the top half of your body to one side twice and then twice to the other side.

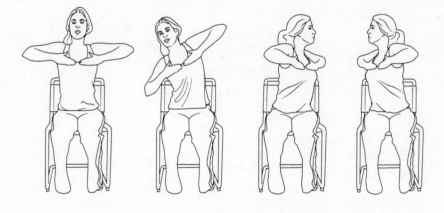

MORE SERIOUS PROBLEMS

Sometimes more serious problems crop up in pregnancy, and you may need to ask to be referred to a physiotherapist.

Pregnancy-related Pelvic Girdle Pain (was called Symphysis Pubis Dysfunction or SPD)

The pelvis is a ring of three bones which are held together by very strong ligaments. The bones meet to form three 'fixed' joints – one in the middle of the front (the symphysis pubis) and at each side of the bottom of the spine (the sacro-iliac joints). Normally these joints are not designed to allow movement.

As soon as you become pregnant, you produce a hormone (appropriately called relaxin) which, amongst other things, allows the ligaments that keep the pelvic bones together to loosen, in preparation for birth. The ligaments sometimes loosen too much, and the joints between the pelvic bones become unstable. There is the possibility that you might do a movement which 'jars' your pelvis, and allows the sacro-iliac joint to move by a millimetre or two, which can give you a pretty unpleasant acute pain at the bottom of your spine to one side. Sometimes the joint at the front of your pelvis (symphysis pubis) actually separates slightly. All this is made worse by the increasing weight of the growing baby.

The most common symptom of pelvic girdle pain is pain when you are walking, possibly accompanied by a feeling that your pelvis is not supporting you properly. The pain is felt in the pubis and/or one or both of the sacro-iliac joints. Pain can also occur in the groin, the inner side of the thighs, the hips or the buttocks.

The pain is usually made worse when:

- turning over in bed
- climbing up stairs
- getting dressed
- getting in and out of the car

In other words, any movement which involves standing on one leg or twisting your pelvis.

When is it Most Likely to Start?

At any time from the first trimester onwards. And some women can be fine during their pregnancy, but get the condition immediately or a few days after their baby has been born. It sometimes occurs following a period of immobility, but conversely can follow an unusually busy overactive period or a particular activity such as swimming breaststroke or lifting something incorrectly, which has stressed any of the three pelvic joints.

Is There Any Treatment?

Unfortunately, as there is no way of tightening the ligaments during pregnancy (although a specialist physiotherapist may be able to help your symptoms) there is no treatment that will 'cure' pelvic girdle pain. This holds for any sort of alternative treatment such as reflexology or acupuncture. However, after your baby has been born, your body stops producing relaxin, so the ligaments tighten up and (for the vast majority of women) the symptoms gradually disappear.

So What Can I Do if I Think I've Got it?

The most important thing is to avoid any movement that aggravates the pain, such as standing on one leg.

- Sit on a chair to get dressed.
- Always turn over in bed with a pillow between your knees (see page 152).
- Lift correctly (see page 124).
- If you go swimming, don't swim breaststroke.
- Get a rest (in bed) every day.
- Make sure your midwife knows you have this condition before you go into labour.
- If you have a car with a clutch, make sure your seat is near enough to the steering wheel so you can work the clutch with your foot and ankle only, rather than through your hip with a straight leg.
- Get into and out of a car carefully, especially a low one. Put your bottom onto the seat first and then lift each leg in, one at a time. Getting out means the reverse. Put one leg out onto the pavement, then the other one. Only when you have both feet on the pavement, as opposed to one foot in the car, lean forwards and stand up. All this is much easier if you have a sensible but perhaps boring car as opposed to a low two-seater sports car. If you do have a sporty car, it might be worth considering that in a few months you will have to fix a baby car seat in the back. Will this be possible? Or do you need to think about changing your car to fit in with your new life?

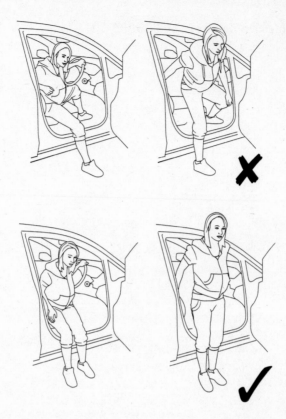

If the pain is severe, go to your GP and ask for a referral to a physiotherapist – ideally one who has specialist training in obstetrics, and is called a Physiotherapist in Women's Health. She will be able to assess you, help you with appropriate exercises and may decide to fit you with a pelvic support belt. Your GP will also be able to prescribe painkillers that are safe to take during pregnancy.

Carpal Tunnel Syndrome in Pregnancy

This is a fairly common condition, resulting from swelling of the tissues around the wrist, which in turn compresses the nerves that supply the hand. It is a real nuisance. Your hand or hands may actually be visibly swollen and your wrists and fingers may feel stiff and clumsy, which makes dressing difficult and cooking positively dangerous. You may have pins and needles, numbness or pain, usually affecting the thumb, index and middle fingers, but sometimes the fourth and fifth fingers instead (or as well). The pain is often worse at night.

What Can You Do?

Ask your GP to refer you to a physiotherapist, who will assess you and possibly supply you with wrist splints. Meanwhile:

- try and reduce activities in which your hand is carried low or exercised, such as shopping, carrying and writing
- wrap a small bag of frozen peas in a wet napkin or tea-towel and put it on the palm side of your wrist for up to 10 minutes
- whenever you can, raise your hands and wrists above your head, which may help to reduce the swelling
- try to sleep with your forearms and hands up on a pillow, again to help move the swelling away from your wrist

All the symptoms should disappear completely in the weeks following delivery.

GENERAL EXERCISE

If you are someone who regularly goes to the gym, you will probably want to continue during your pregnancy. This is fine but now may be the time to start cutting back a little. Exercise is good as long as you don't overdo it – to my mind twice a week at the gym is quite enough when you are pregnant. After all, walking is perfectly good exercise, although you will probably need to walk more slowly than your usual non-pregnant pace.

Don't go to the gym at all if:

- your baby isn't growing as well as he should be
- you are seriously underweight yourself, and you panic if you can't exercise regularly
- you have placenta praevia (see page 50) or any vaginal bleeding

If you regularly visit the gym, your weekly exercise time should tot up to about two-thirds of what you were doing before pregnancy. And you should not exercise to the point of a racing heart – for most women, 140 beats a minute is quite fast enough. This bit is important – muscles that are worked really hard need more oxygen, so there is a danger of your blood supply being diverted from the placenta in order to feed your muscles – this is obviously not in the interests of your baby. The same general principle applies to exercise classes: you can continue them as long as your teacher knows you are pregnant and moderates your cardiac output as well as adjusting any active abdominal exercises to take your pregnancy into account.

On the other hand, if you take no regular exercise but you feel pregnancy is the time to begin, your best bet is to book into specific pregnancy exercise classes and/or take to the pool. Being fit won't make you more likely to have a straightforward labour. There is no evidence that physical fitness has any effect at all on the length and type of labour you will experience. (Life's not fair, as we all know.) However, women who are fit will have more stamina for a long labour, and fit women also tend to recover physically and heal more quickly following childbirth.

Avoid 'impact' exercises such as running or jogging and

'bouncy' classes involving leaping around. You don't want to put a strain on already loosened ligaments, especially those that support your uterus. And listen to your body – if you feel pain anywhere, or tired, dizzy or nauseous, stop! Obviously! Now is not the time to try and increase your exercise tolerance. Keep up your fluid levels when exercising, and unlike in your previous non-pregnant life, don't try to resist the carbohydrates you crave afterwards. You (and your baby) need them.

Swimming

Again, if you are a regular swimmer, I would suggest you cut down on the weekly lengths you were swimming before you were pregnant – and swim more slowly. Swimming is an ideal exercise to take up during pregnancy as it will mobilise your spine and joints as well as generally working most muscle groups without jarring your joints.

However, cut out breaststroke if:

- you find the front of your pelvis (symphysis pubis) feels sore or unstable afterwards (see Pelvic Girdle Pain, page 129)
- you notice you have slight low backache after a swim

Pilates

As long as your teacher knows you are pregnant, Pilates classes are a great way of exercising groups of muscles without putting stress on your joints. The exercises will, for example, work your underneath corset abdominal muscle group, without damaging the recti muscles (see above) and keep your bottom muscles toned. And Pilates teachers know about the importance of exercising your pelvic floor muscles.

Yoga

Most women tell me that they really enjoy yoga classes during pregnancy, but again, it's best to ensure that they are specifically designed for pregnant women. You don't want to do too much joint stretching as it will put a strain on your already looser ligaments. If anything aches after the class, work out which movement may have been responsible and avoid doing it again.

Other Sports

Don't go scuba diving – it is not good news for your baby because of his oxygen needs. Otherwise – although now is clearly not the time to take up bungee jumping, kick boxing or judo – how long you continue activities such as horse riding, skiing or cycling very much depends on how experienced and competent you are. From my experience, women vary enormously as to how long they continue these activities. **But it is worth bearing in mind that when you are pregnant your sense of balance is not as good as it is when you are not pregnant** – and it would seem sensible to stop as soon as your confidence in this respect drops a little.

Impact sports, such as tennis, squash and golf, make you more likely to damage a joint (due to the loose ligaments). Although it is unlikely that any sports injury will damage your baby, there is a theoretical risk of a hard ball hitting him. By the second trimester, as he is lying above your pelvic bones, he is not protected by them. But this is a common-sense theoretical danger. There can't really be a rule – yet again, this must be left to the individual sensible woman who is listening to her body. You obviously don't want to put your baby at risk – therefore you will decide when is the right time to stop.

CHAPTER 9

pregnancy-related irritations and changes in your body

The following are the most usual worries and 'grumbles' that women bring up during antenatal classes – and it helps to know what is normal during pregnancy. Some of you might be lucky enough to find that you love being pregnant and have very few of these complaints!

Putting on Weight

The 'average' weight gain in pregnancy is around 28 lb (2 stone or 13 kg). But of course not all women are average and, quite honestly, women vary enormously when it comes to how much weight they put on during pregnancy. A lucky few seem to gain weight only where the bump is, and from behind no-one would know they were pregnant. But some of you will find that the pounds start to pile on as soon as you become pregnant – partly because you are starving hungry all the time and partly because you seem to suffer from fluid retention. Let's face it, no-one actually wants to put on masses of weight during their pregnancy, and if you find that this is happening to you, you secretly worry that you will never lose it. This worry is not helped when girlfriends imply the same.

You all know what a balanced diet is – stick to this, but bear in mind you need to eat roughly an extra 300 calories a day while pregnant. There is plenty of advice out there as to what you should eat but if you are feeling really uncertain, look at the advice from the Food Standards Agency (www.eatwell.gov.uk). As long as you are not living on a diet of chips and doughnuts, try not to worry too much about extra weight gain and relax into the size that you are at present. If you have put on more weight than you 'should', you can, and will if you want to, return to your pre-pregnancy size after you have had your baby.

WHAT ON EARTH CAN I WEAR?

Some women seem to sail through pregnancy looking as gorgeous as always, with just a neat bump in the correct place to show anyone who might notice that they are expecting a baby. If you are tall and slim you may be one of these lucky few, so you can skip this section. Tall, long-waisted women have more room to accommodate their growing baby (which is why people helpfully remark 'Isn't your baby small') and may well get away with not going anywhere near custom-made maternity clothes.

If you are short you are more likely to have a greater problem, especially if you have also been blessed with large breasts. When pregnant, your bump tends to look bigger than the bump of a tall woman (and yes, people helpfully remark 'Aren't you big') simply because you have less room to accommodate him. The baby you are carrying may seem to have taken you over completely. This, coupled with large breasts that have increased by a couple of cup sizes, means it can be very difficult not to look completely spherical.

Just buying regular tops in XXL size is not as obvious an answer as it may seem, as T-shirts and sweaters in this size are also made with long arms, which tend to be irritating. Although the tops of your arms may get fatter, your arms won't become longer. (That is the drawback about thinking you can wear your husband's shirts – they are fine for casual wear over trousers with the cuffs turned back, but usually won't fit under a suit jacket.)

If you have to buy a work suit when you are still only four months pregnant, *do not underestimate how much bigger you are going to get*. Unfortunately, you are not having to deal just with a growing waistline – for many of us, it is a bit of a shock to find that as well as the baby, several other bits (hips, thighs, bottom, chest and upper arms) become larger, and assistants in maternity clothes shops are sometimes totally unrealistic about this. At the end of your pregnancy, you certainly do not want to be squeezing yourself into an expensive work suit you bought four months ago that now feels too tight. As well as wearing clothes that look OK, they must be comfortable. Believe me, you will feel pretty uncomfortable in any case, without having the tops of your trouser legs cutting into your groin when you are sitting down. So think ahead generously.

Before you go anywhere near a shop that sells maternity clothes, bear the following points in mind:

- Only a lucky few put on just the recommended amount of weight (see above).
- Unfortunately, extra weight seems to appear around your bottom and thighs as well as your tummy.
- From around 28–31 weeks your ribcage expands and continues to do so in order to accommodate the baby, so any shirt or jacket must allow for this.
- Your tummy may feel itchy, so anything covering it needs to be cotton rather than nylon, if possible.
- Don't think you will want to wear anything you wore when you were pregnant after you have had the baby – you won't.

For work, dark trouser suits are probably the smartest option. It is easier to go for trousers, as they cope with the tights and shoe problem (see opposite). The jacket *must be long enough to cover at least some of your bottom* (which will not be the bottom you know). The same applies to waistcoats, if you wear them. The trousers need to be roomy enough (roomier than you might think), not only around the waist and bum area, but also at the tops of the thighs. Unfortunately, this is where you also tend to put on weight, and where the baby will be hanging over when you sit down. And at the end of pregnancy, when your expensive maternity trousers slip down over your belly, it's worth trying a pair of men's braces.

Bear in mind that many women frequently feel hot and sweaty when they are pregnant, so be wary of buying tops in wool. At the end of pregnancy it is also usual to find it difficult to eat without slopping food down your bump (no, really), so a pale-coloured cashmere number might not be practical in any case.

You may be able to get away with one suit, a waistcoat type of

·garment and several different T-shirts. There is, however, an area of your body which actually looks better when you are pregnant – your cleavage. Go for it. Avoid T-shirts with a high round neck and stick to those with a V-neck or shirts with a collar or front opening. A collar and open buttons at the neck will take the eye away from the expanse of belly.

If yours is a summer pregnancy, the joy of a dress without tights is obvious – there is nothing round your tummy area, and if you have pale legs you can safely use fake tan and get away without wearing tights. Many maternity dresses (apart from being an expensive item for such a short time) often have the knack of making pregnant women look either demure or mumsy. High-street non-maternity shops are usually worth taking a look in.

Tights

Tights when pregnant are nearly always unsatisfactory. Some people find maternity tights (which have an enormous top to stretch over your tummy) more comfortable than ordinary tights worn rolled up under your tummy. Most women find that neither option is perfect, especially if the tights have to be worn all day. This is coupled with the normal pregnancy problem of an itchy tummy and restless legs (see page 145) – both of which are exacerbated by man-made fibres. If you are not able to go bare-legged, most women find it more comfortable to wear trousers and socks.

Shoes

Guess what else gets bigger – yes, your feet! (The extra weight you are carrying, coupled with the hormone relaxin, usually allows the many ligaments between the bones in your feet to stretch.) Shoes worn during pregnancy will not be wearable after you have had the baby. Again, if yours is a summer pregnancy, the pros of wearing flip-flops are obvious.

It is a bad idea to wear heels for longer than an hour or so – you are much more at risk of developing low backache (see page 121). As you are also at risk of losing your balance and falling over when you are pregnant, your shoes must support you properly. Therefore you are left with a small choice of shoes that are flat, comfortable and preferably contain some elastic. These are what are called sensible shoes – you might think this could be another reason for getting into trousers so you can cover them up.

Bras

As soon as you are pregnant, you are likely to notice that your breasts feel sensitive (so much that it can be rather unpleasant) and start to become bigger. At around the three-month mark you will probably need to buy a larger bra – usually bigger by one or two cup sizes and one chest size.

This new bra should see you through to about 28 weeks, but you may then find your ribcage continues to get wider, although with any luck, your breasts will stay more or less the same size. From 28 weeks, don't get seduced into buying yet another new bra if the one you are wearing is too tight but the cup size is OK – you can buy bra extenders in the haberdashery department of John Lewis and other department stores. These extenders just hook on to your existing bra hooks (no sewing involved) to give you more room round your back.

Incidentally, if none of the above applies to you, and your breasts just remain the same, don't panic – this *doesn't mean* there will be a problem with breastfeeding later.

Underwired Bras

I have never quite understood the tut-tuttings or dire warnings when it comes to wearing underwired bras during pregnancy. Presumably, if the underwire sits on the breast rather than the ribcage, there is a theoretical danger that the wire will compress and damage a milk duct (which is needed to carry milk to your baby) after you have given birth. But if the underwire is sitting in the correct place (under rather than on the breast) I cannot see what the problem might be. I have never come across anyone who has had difficulties breastfeeding because a bra wire damaged her milk ducts during her pregnancy... If you want (or need) to wear an underwired bra, do so, but it might be sensible to just check at the end of the day that there is no wire mark on your actual breast.

Nursing/feeding Bras

These are bras (without an underwire but much prettier than they used to be!) designed for breastfeeding. The cup opens at the front (by zip or hook) so that you can easily feed your baby without having to take off half your clothes. Even if you know you are definitely not going to breastfeed, it is worth buying one of these. When your milk 'comes in' a few days after you give birth (and the milk will arrive even if you don't put your baby to the breast) you will need something fairly powerful and comfortable to contain your large and tender breasts.

On your list of 'things to do' must be to get a nursing bra well before your baby is due – around 34–36 weeks. It's probably best to get fitted by a specialist bra fitter, but they are trained not to fit pregnant women before they are 36–38 weeks. Quite honestly this is really not practical, bearing in mind that a quarter of babies will have been born at 38 weeks, and you will be unlikely to feel like struggling up to a department store when you are 37 weeks pregnant. The simplest way to pre-empt any difficulty is to always tell the assistant that you are 37 weeks pregnant.

Some of you will buy nursing bras on the internet. Although this clearly saves trailing off to a shop to be fitted, it may not be quite as good an option as it seems, since you will have a serious problem if the bra doesn't actually fit when your milk comes in! But if you have already bought one, try it on when you are 35 or more weeks pregnant. The nursing bra should be on the very last hook round your ribcage (as your ribcage will start to get smaller again once your baby is born) and with the cups roomy enough to allow an increase by up to two more breast sizes (yes, really!). When your milk comes in three or four days after your baby has been born, the increase in your breast size can be extremely dramatic for a week or so.

Cramp

No-one knows exactly why pregnant women suffer from cramp in their calf muscles. One theory is that the cause is low levels of minerals, such as calcium and magnesium, so some obstetricians prescribe supplement tablets, which seem to help some women, though not all. Another theory is that cramp is caused by the pressure of your baby on nerves or on blood vessels in your pelvis, causing a decrease in the return of blood from your legs, which is why women are prone to leg cramps at night. But whatever the cause, most women suffer from this really annoying problem, particularly just as they have finally drifted off to sleep.

Before going to bed, try sitting or lying with your legs higher than your pelvis. Then waggle your feet up and down and round in a circle as vigorously as possible. You need to do this exercise for about 10 minutes or until your calf muscles start to ache a bit! This may prevent or at least improve the night cramps.

If you do wake up in the night with excruciating leg cramp, the one thing that gets rid of it is to get out of bed, put the foot of the affected leg flat on the floor in front of you and bend the leg, taking the knee forwards and putting all your weight on the affected leg.

The good news is that as soon as you have had your baby, the cramps will disappear.

Restless Legs

This problem is exactly as described – you find it difficult to keep your legs still and you may feel you need to repeatedly massage them. It is a well-recognised problem and not uncommon, occurring whether you are pregnant or not, though often pregnancy is the first time you might suffer from it. If so, it usually clears up when you have had your baby. Going to the theatre or cinema can be a nightmare as you find your legs will just not stay still. It is another problem when you try to get some sleep at night.

I'm not sure that there is anything you can do to prevent this, but try having a hot bath in the evening, followed by giving your legs a good massage with body lotion. (Wearing man-made fibres such as tights seems to make things worse.) Bear in mind that you may find your restless legs more of a problem if you are overtired and/or stressed, so it's worth monitoring whether you are more likely to have a bout of restless legs after a very full day, rather than a day when you have had a rest. If this is the case, you will want to cut things back a bit.

Itching

At the end of the day, you can't wait to get home and take your clothes off! Your stretched tummy itches, and usually feels much worse if you have to wear tights over, rather than under, your bump. The waistband of skirts and trousers become really irritating. This is normal, and rubbing in aqueous cream (bought over the counter from chemists) should help. However, *if you find you are itching seriously all over*, especially over the palms of your hands and feet (as opposed to just your tummy area), *you need to report this to your midwife* as soon as possible. This can be a sign of a potentially serious (but very rare) condition called cholestasis of pregnancy, which affects your liver, and occasionally can be a threat to your baby. It can be diagnosed by a blood test.

Heartburn

The hormone progesterone relaxes the smooth muscle of your gut and slows its activity in pregnancy. It also means that the valve at the bottom of your oesophagus is less able to prevent acid regurgitation from your stomach, which is why so many pregnant women suffer from heartburn. You can buy liquid or tablets, such as Gaviscon and Rennies, from a chemist. If things are really bad, ask your chemist to give you some magnesium trisilicate (Mist. Mag. Trisilicate) – a rather heavy chalky substance that pretty well always does the trick. It's probably best to avoid actual drugs which you can buy over the counter, such as ranitidine (Zantac) and so on, until you have talked to your GP. The manufacturers advise caution with their use in pregnancy, though there is actually no positive evidence of harm to the baby in humans.

Most women find it best to eat smaller, more frequent meals, and some women find it helps to have a yoghurt or some ice cream before going to bed. Sometimes the only way to cope with heartburn at night is by sleeping in an almost upright position, with the help of lots of pillows or a V-shaped pillow.

Feeling Sick (see also Chapter 1)

The uterus rises upwards as pregnancy advances, and by around 32 weeks nearly reaches the stomach, pushing it against the diaphragm and stopping it being able to expand as much as before you became pregnant. It's often a disaster for you if your husband works long hours and you have to eat supper at 9pm – you are absolutely starving so you bolt down your food, and as your stomach can't expand as efficiently, you feel pretty sick or actually throw up. Tackle it in the same way as heartburn with frequent small meals, especially a 'high tea' snack early evening. Things get better if your baby engages at around 36–37 weeks (see Chapter 10).

Cravings

Some women develop a desire for rather strange foods – commonly highly spiced, pickled things as well as chocolate (of course) and other sweet foods, and at the other end of the spectrum, a need to eat ice cubes. An urge to lick coal is not usual, but has been known to happen! Go with your cravings – although they can be extraordinary, as far as I know no-one has had any craving that damaged her baby.

Conversely, you may find some tastes and smells are now hard to take or find you have a funny taste in your mouth and have 'gone off' things such as coffee or alcohol, which in your previous life were part of your staple diet. In this instance you are probably fortunate – you tend to 'go off' things that aren't good for your baby anyway. Clever Mother Nature (see Chapter 7).

Constipation

This is another annoying problem for most women – once again it's caused by the release of extra progesterone during pregnancy, which slows down your digestive system, or rather the gut transit time. There's no magic solution, apart from the obvious remedies of keeping your fluid levels up and eating plenty of fruit and fibre, especially kiwi fruit and figs. If you are taking iron tablets, these can make things worse – keep changing the iron preparation until you find one that makes you the least constipated as different preparations affect women differently.

Varicose Veins

You may notice to your horror that you are developing bluish-purple strings of varicose veins, usually on the lower part of your legs, and sometimes around your vulva. They are swollen veins caused by the heavy uterus blocking the return flow of blood from your legs and lower abdomen. The veins during pregnancy are also more 'relaxed' by progesterone, and this, coupled with the normal increase in blood volume, adds to the problem. They are very common in pregnancy. If you find the veins ache, it's important that you don't stand for any longer than necessary, and it will help to wear support tights. Don't wear socks (especially pop socks) with tight elastic round one part of your leg, and try not to sit with your legs crossed.

Vulval varicose veins can ache terribly – it will help if you lie down at some stage during the day with a pillow under your bottom (so your pelvis is higher than your tummy) and do your pelvic floor exercise (see page 119). This should help the pooling blood move along the veins.

Do not panic – all types of varicose veins usually disappear, or at least fade after delivery. It is usually a hereditary problem – if your parents have varicose veins, you may well develop them as well. You absolutely **don't** develop varicose veins because you have failed to use some sort of special cream, not had enough reflexology or have been wearing unsuitable shoes.

Piles (Haemorrhoids)

These are simply varicose veins (see above) of the anal area, and they can sometimes bleed (bright red rather than dark red blood), itch or be painful. If you discover that you have developed them, you may find it embarrassing to talk about, not to mention the fact you are likely to feel incredibly geriatric. It's worth buying an over-the-counter topical ointment and trying to increase the fibre in your diet. Again, they will disappear when you have had your baby. They don't need an operation.

Stretch Marks

At the end of pregnancy you may get undressed in front of a mirror and see – shock, horror! – purple lines running down underneath your tummy, and possibly your thighs and breasts too. You will probably think, 'Oh my God – how desperately unattractive. I'll never be able to wear a bikini again.' Try not to panic – they will (almost) disappear when you have had your baby, and certainly they will fade to a pale colour that will not be noticeable to anyone else. Three out of five women get stretch marks during pregnancy, and again, they tend to be a hereditary problem. Some people simply inherit less elasticity in their skin than others. **NO creams can prevent stretch marks** – in spite of what the blurb on the jar may claim.

Pigmentation

When standing in front of the mirror with no clothes on you might also notice a brown line running vertically up the front of your tummy, crossing your navel. The brown line is called the linea nigra. (If you don't notice it during pregnancy, you will see it after you have had your baby.) This, again, is quite normal – and it will fade during the months after your baby has been born. The pregnancy pigmentation will also make your nipples and the areola (area round the nipples) look darker. And it can affect your face, darkening the skin around your cheeks, nose and eyes to give a 'butterfly' appearance. (It's called chloasma, or perhaps rather ominously, 'the mask of pregnancy'.) If you notice that you are affected, the sun will make it much more pronounced, so be careful to protect your face in the summer.

Puffy Ankles, Feet and Hands

At around 30 weeks onwards, it is usual for women to find their ankles and fingers swell slightly. Swollen ankles and feet are nothing to worry about **as long as your blood pressure is normal** and there is no protein in your urine – things always checked at your antenatal appointments in case of pre-eclampsia (see page 48). If you suddenly swell up, go and get your blood pressure checked. It will help the swelling of your ankles and feet to subside if you manage to lie down for an hour during the daytime. It will also help if you can prop up your legs at the end of the day, by putting your feet on a cushion on a chair. Then, while you are watching television, move your feet vigorously up and down and then in circles, so your calf muscles start to ache – as in trying to prevent cramp (see above).

Swollen fingers, on their own, are again common in pregnancy. Most women find they have to put their rings aside at around this time, but are sometimes reluctant to take off their wedding ring. If it is getting tight, it's very important to do so – fingers can swell dramatically at 36 weeks, and this sometimes means that a tight wedding ring has to be cut off because there is a danger it can impair the circulation to your finger. **Check your rings frequently** – if it looks as though there might be a problem getting them off, take them off now! If there is already a problem, don't panic. Try putting your hand in ice, wind cotton round and round your finger to reduce its thickness and try to slide the ring over this with the help of some washing-up liquid.

Teeth

It used to be said that you lose a tooth for each baby you have – but this is an old wives' tale. However, make sure you visit your dentist, because if there is any work that needs to be done, it is best to sort it out before you have your baby – going to the dentist is not easy when you have a small baby in tow. On the NHS, there is no charge for women who are pregnant and this continues until their baby is 12 months old.

It is perfectly OK to have fillings (and X-rays if necessary), as long as your dentist knows that you are pregnant.

Bleeding gums are common during pregnancy (due to hormonal changes). If this is a nuisance when you are brushing your teeth, it might be worth trying a softer toothbrush. Your dentist might also suggest you see the hygienist.

Blocked Nose and Snoring

The general increase in tissue fluid in pregnancy often results in your having what seems like a permanently blocked nose, and this in turn can make you snore at night. Horrors! And your husband will undoubtedly let you know. Beconase nasal spray is OK to use occasionally, which means not every four hours every day (it does say on the leaflet that you should consult your pharmacist or doctor), and will get rid of your blocked nose. Needless to say, this little problem will also disappear after you have had your baby.

Tired and Irritable

This is a very common issue – many women say they feel exhausted and fed up in the evenings – and their husbands often take the brunt ('He has absolutely no idea what it's like to be pregnant ALL of the time') (see Chapter 14). You may also find that you are clumsy and forgetful and do odd things. (One woman reported she put a tea bag in the dishwasher instead of a washing tablet.) Go with it – all of the above is normal!

Feeling Light-headed, Dizzy or Faint

When I'm taking an antenatal class, there's often someone outside the door feeling faint and having a cup of sugared tea with my secretary. Again, it's a rather embarrassing problem (especially in the office) but not unusual. It's rare to actually faint, but if you do, you will need to consider whether you should stop driving for the time being. Keep some sugar-laden stuff in your handbag to eat, and if you start to feel hot and light-headed, get up (slowly) sooner rather than later, and head off to an open window.

Can't Sleep at Night

As soon as you attempt to get a rest during the day – perhaps dutifully trying to do what I've suggested – you find you can't sleep during the night. And you think, 'This is ridiculous – as soon as I've

started to sleep during the day, I find I'm sleeping badly at night.'
This is honestly NOT due to the nap during the day!

Most women don't sleep well at night after 34 weeks. I sometimes wonder if nature is getting them braced for the fact that
actually they're not going to sleep very well during the night for the
few months after birth… It is common to find that your mind starts
racing as soon as you lie down, and you may find you are fretting
about something really trivial such as a conversation you had with
someone earlier in the day. You may also find you are thinking about
your mother… All this may seem most peculiar, but is normal and
really common.

Your difficulty in sleeping well at night may be made worse by the
fact that during pregnancy it is more difficult for you to regulate your
body temperature. You find you are suddenly terribly hot at night
and MUST HAVE SOME AIR. At the same time your partner is
freezing cold and really fed up with you tossing and turning, and
getting in and out of bed for repeated pees. Such is married bliss.

Finding a Comfortable Sleeping Position

You may have been told that under no circumstances should you lie
on your back to sleep, as you will starve your baby of oxygen. So you
go to bed, carefully settle yourself on one side only to wake in the
night and find you are lying flat on your back. Panic – 'Oh my God,
now I've brain-damaged my baby.' But don't panic any more – you
won't have brain-damaged your baby. As it happens, most pregnant
women find they can't lie on their back at the end of pregnancy
because it makes them feel dizzy and faint. This is because the weight
of their baby presses against the large vein (vena cava) that transports
blood to the heart, resulting in the heart being able to pump rather

less blood to the head. Feeling dizzy is your body's way of telling you that there is a potential problem, so you automatically turn over. But if you want to settle yourself to sleep on your back when you are more than 24 weeks pregnant, it's a good idea to put a pillow or foam wedge under your right hip; this will be enough to shift your baby off the blood vessels and avoid the problem.

You may also be told to 'lie only on your right side' as this will supply your baby with more oxygen and encourage him to get into a good position for the start of labour. There is no evidence to support this but babies are often more comfortable if you lie on one side or the other, and this changes. One way or another (by wriggling, for instance), your baby will let you know which side you can, and therefore should, lie on. You may find that some nights you and he can't get comfortable on one particular side and other nights it will be the other side. As he changes his position, you will find that you also want to alter yours.

Extra pillows in bed help most women feel more comfortable – you will probably need to buy at least a couple more. But don't begrudge this – extra pillows will also be essential once you have had your baby as you will find you spend many, many hours feeding your baby in bed. It's odd how we are quite happy to shell out God knows how much on an Italian/French babygro, but rather resent buying a couple of extra pillows. Squidgy polyester-type ones are probably the most useful, and they can be washed if necessary.

You will need a thick pillow to go between your knees, and a thinner pillow to put between the bump and the mattress (see diagram). Keeping the thick pillow between your knees will also make you keep your knees together when you turn over in the night, and will protect your unstable pelvis. This is vital if you have pelvic girdle pain/SPD (see Chapter 8). The thin pillow will support the weight of the uterus, which will help prevent the ligaments from being overstretched.

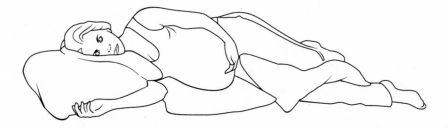

One other problem is that many women find that the hip they are lying on becomes very sore. (Interestingly, when I worked as an antenatal expert on a website, this was a really common problem raised by pregnant women.) I still don't know any brilliant solution to this, but many of you have said that folding up a single duvet, making it into a sort of nest and lying on it helps! Other women have reported that buying a mattress topper has helped.

Vaginal Discharge

This is normal during pregnancy – all the time – and some of you will find you have to wear a panty liner every day. If the discharge is clear and doesn't smell, all is OK, but if it looks brown, yellow or green, smells unpleasant, is associated with an itch or hurts when you pee, contact your GP.

Thrush (Candida)

This is a yeast infection of the vagina, and nothing to do with not washing yourself properly. Although it's seriously irritating to you, it is not a serious condition in itself and does not harm your baby.

The infection produces a whitish discharge and usually some redness, but perhaps much more importantly to you usually makes your crutch itch. Some women are more prone to this than others, and those of you who have had this before will know that if you have to take a course of antibiotics, you are very likely to develop thrush afterwards. It will also tend to appear when the weather is hot and during pregnancy (because of high levels of oestrogen in your blood). If you don't have time to collect a free prescription from your GP, you can now buy over-the-counter pessaries and creams, which are OK to use when pregnant (but don't take any oral treatment unless this is prescribed). Obviously, wear cotton pants and avoid tights.

And at the End of Pregnancy...

You will have real trouble cutting your toenails, shaving your legs and putting on your socks. Keep your sense of humour – you are not alone!

CHAPTER 10

last lap of pregnancy

YOUR STATE OF MIND!

From about 36 weeks, pregnancy loses its bloom for many women, and you may be beginning to feel that you have had enough. It is worth mentioning that it is not that unusual (but rarely admitted) for some women to find they feel a little 'depressed'. A few women in my last antenatal class have said things like, 'If anyone else says to me "Aren't you excited?" I think I might say something terrible, such as "No! I'm bloody fed up and I don't think I want it now."' Although this emotion isn't by any means what everyone feels, when a woman verbalises such an extreme view, I notice that the other women all nod their heads sympathetically, and some offer examples of similar feelings in themselves. No-one looks shocked!

It might be worth viewing mild antenatal depression as a sign that you are well-prepared for a dramatically different life ahead. Feeling flat at the end of pregnancy is not an indication that you are more likely to suffer from postnatal depression. From my experience, it's the women who anticipate the joys of blissful motherhood – perhaps imagining their baby is going to be sleeping (clothed in really cute gear) in a Moses basket all day – who are much more at risk.

You may also find that you are making what seems to be an awful lot of lists, and ticking things off every day. In a way it's quite a difficult time because you really don't know if you have another six weeks to go or perhaps only one…so planning your social life isn't easy. You can have your baby any time after 37 weeks – just as you can be 10 days overdue.

YOUR BABY DOES NOT STOP MOVING AT THE END OF PREGNANCY

Apart from everyone confidently predicting whether you are carrying a boy or a girl and how big your baby is going to be, some girlfriends will tell you that your baby stops moving at the end of pregnancy. **This is absolutely not true.** Babies never stop moving for more than a few hours, although the nature of the movements might feel different in late pregnancy because he has less space. You can often elicit a movement by giving your baby a 'push' with your hand or eating sugar, such as a cup of sweet tea. But if you are worried or unsure about his movements, **go straight to the labour ward so your baby can be monitored**. No member of staff in the labour ward will ever make you feel stupid for 'bothering' them. This, again, is an issue of trusting your instincts – if you have any niggling worries go to hospital.

WHAT TO BUY AND PACK FOR LABOUR

It's wise to try and buy everything you need by the time you are 37 weeks pregnant. Although you can certainly pack your cases whilst you are in labour, you probably won't want to drive off to the chemist to buy sanitary pads – or have to send your husband. The following list has been compiled from the suggestions made by hundreds of women whom I have taken for antenatal classes over the years and who have been kind enough to update me on what they needed. This means that not everyone will use everything on it.

Most women will deliver their baby in a delivery room on the labour ward and are transferred to a postnatal ward afterwards. There is very little room for luggage in hospitals, and the less clobber you bring in the better – you certainly won't want to be dragging round a large suitcase. If you are not having your baby privately (in which case you sometimes deliver in your own room), it makes sense to have two separate lightweight bags – one for the labour ward and another for your stay in the postnatal ward. The latter can be left in the car and collected by your partner later.

Labour Ward Bag

You will need to pack the following:

Your hospital notes – if you, rather than your hospital, are in charge of them

A nightdress
The good news is that you do not have to deliver your baby with nothing on your top half (in spite of what you may see on rather

alarming TV birth programmes where every mother seems to be completely naked). Most women wear their own nightdress or a large T-shirt when they are admitted, although many women change into a hospital gown if they have an epidural, simply because they do up at the back. When you have had your baby, you will change back into your own nightdress again.

A lightweight dressing gown and a pair of flip-flops (or similar)
In case you want to walk up and down the hospital corridor during early labour, and/or walk to the shower or loo when you've had your baby.

A spongebag
Containing: flannel, soap, toothbrush, mouthwash (you may develop a very dry mouth), hairbrush and small towel. Possibly lipsalve and a scrunchie to tie back your hair.

A watch with a second hand
This is so you can time the contractions. Although there is likely to be a clock in the delivery room, some women have said that they were totally thrown to find it wasn't working!

iPod and speakers or similar
If you have a long labour, you might want music. But you won't want earphones because you will need to talk and listen to your midwife.

A couple of sanitary pads and a pair of disposable or old pants
Most hospitals will give you a sanitary pad when you have delivered

your baby, but there have been reports of you being expected to provide your own. And a sanitary pad is useless without a pair of pants to hold it in place!

Camera

This is not for your partner to take a photo of your baby's head crowning, but to take a photo of you and your baby as soon as possible after his birth. It will be very precious years down the line.

Glasses or spare contact lens if you use them

Some women find that contact lenses are just not comfortable when they are in labour.

Nappy, vest and swaddling sheet

Two extra pillows with coloured pillow cases (leave in car)

There is a possibility that you will need more pillows than the hospital provides on the labour ward. In any case, for an overnight stay in hospital, your own pillow is a real bonus! A coloured pillow case (as opposed to a white one) will mean you will be less likely to leave it behind.

A list of names for your husband to ring

As you are in organisation mode, it seems only sensible to make a list of the essential people whom you will want him to phone when you have had your baby. Your own mother should be top of the list.

Food and fluid

Possibly for your partner when you are in labour in case he does not have time to leave the hospital, but definitely for you afterwards. You won't want to eat during the active stage of labour, but once you have had your baby you will be starving – and you will want sugar!

And anything else your antenatal teacher suggests
She, of course, will know the hospitals in your area, whereas I am only familiar with London hospitals.

Postnatal Ward Bag

One or two spare nightdresses
Women can find they are very sweaty after giving birth, so you will probably need to think about getting through two per day.

Nursing bra
This will be needed if your breasts are uncomfortable without support, and definitely once your milk comes in on the third or fourth day.

Breast pads
These are disposable leak-proof pads, which sit between your breasts and your bra. You can buy them from a chemist. Not everyone needs them – but some of you will find you leak colostrum or milk.

More sanitary pads

Extra snack food
You will continue to be hungry and hospital food is often not

enough. You will also be anxious to keep your bowels ticking over, so it might be worth taking some of your own breakfast muesli and some apples, as well as biscuits.

Notebook and pen

Don't be alarmed to find that you are pretty 'brain-dead' immediately after birth and can't remember anything. It's helpful to be able to write down the last time your baby fed and which breast he finished on, so you know this is the breast to start on next time.

Mobile phone and charger (if mobiles are allowed)

The charger is the most common item that women tell me they forget!

Tissues/loo paper

Coloured towels

Swimming towels are good as they dry quickly and, again, because of their colour you are less likely to leave them behind. You might want to take in a small hand towel to use as a bathmat.

Disposable nappies and a muslin (for mopping up baby sick)

Spare baby clothes and swaddling sheet

Your baby will only need to wear a vest or nightgown (rather than a babygro) as hospitals are very hot.

Baby soap or aqueous cream and large cotton wool balls

Baby nail scissors/clippers or emery board

A couple of carrier bags
For dirty clothes and rubbish!

Put out at Home for Your Husband to Bring when He Collects You

- baby car seat
- a bag in the car seat containing:
  - fresh clothes for your baby to come home in, including a shawl/blanket and baby hat
  - shawl or pashmina for you, especially if you arrived at the hospital without a jacket

BIRTH PLAN

Some hospitals suggest pregnant women write a birth plan to give to the midwife when they are in labour. Paradoxically, rather than finding this reassuring, I've noticed that it seems to cause most of you quite a bit of stress! 'What should I put?' Hopefully, none of you will have a rigid birth plan – we've been through all the reasons for that (see page 30). But in some ways, a birth plan can also alert staff they may be looking after someone who is going to be horribly upset if her ideal birth doesn't go to plan. I would preface whatever you put down with the words – 'an open mind', then add whatever you would ideally like, such as 'an early epidural' or 'ideally a natural birth' and so on. You might want to add thoughts or worries about when your baby is born, such as: 'I would like/hate my baby to be delivered onto my tummy.'

STAYING NEAR HOME!

When we book women in for antenatal classes, we always plan to finish their course when they are no more than 37 weeks pregnant. Even so, it still often happens that someone has already unexpectedly had their baby by the last class.

From 37 weeks, you are likely to find that you are not only tired and vulnerable but also don't really want to stray too far from home. If your partner is away, you may be alarmed to find that you miss him and feel a bit uneasy on your own at night. As your self-confidence is rather low, you will often feel you don't want to let your husband or friends down by bowing out of something such as a previously accepted wedding invitation or a weekend with either set of parents. (I can't tell you how many women I have taken for classes who have ended up having their baby a couple of weeks early in a local hospital while staying with their in-laws!) So the message is – think carefully if you have accepted an invitation to a function that is more than an hour or so away. Do you really want to go? If you do, put your labour bags in the car boot, and if you don't, trust your instincts and have the confidence to stay at home.

IS THE BABY ENGAGED?

At the end of pregnancy you may wonder anxiously when your baby is going to engage or 'drop'. When your baby engages, his head moves lower down into your pelvis – you will know when this happens because it will feel as though your baby's head is literally starting to appear between your legs – and you now need to go to the loo every hour. But at the same time, you are able to breathe more easily.

Babies usually engage some time from 36 weeks onwards. Fifty per cent of first-time mothers find their babies engage any time after 38 weeks, though some don't engage at all. Second- or third-time mothers find that their babies engage later or don't engage until they actually go into labour. If your baby engages it is a good sign, because this increases the chance of you having a straightforward labour. But if your baby doesn't engage it's not necessarily a 'bad' sign!

OH, IT'S BREECH!

From 34 weeks, the majority of babies are lying head down – and remain in this position ready for birth. By 37 weeks nearly all first-time mothers' babies are in this position. Around 4 per cent of babies are lying in the breech position – bottom down – at 37 weeks, at which point they are unlikely to turn round spontaneously.

Recent studies have shown that breech babies delivered vaginally are at a much higher risk of complications, and most obstetricians are now unwilling to attempt a vaginal breech birth, especially for first-time mothers. So, for most women, if your baby is breech at 34 weeks your midwife is likely to do two things – book you in for a scan to confirm that your baby is definitely breech and then make an appointment for you to see an obstetrician.

Is There Anything I Can Do to Encourage Him to Turn?

You will be told of many ways to help a breech baby 'turn' – ranging from reflexology and acupuncture to lying on your back with your legs up against a wall. Although none of the above will harm your baby, extensive trials have shown that there is essentially nothing a mother can do to encourage her baby to turn!

By the time you are due to see the obstetrician, your baby may have turned and now be head down. Problem solved. But if he hasn't and is still in a breech position, your obstetrician may discuss with you the possibility of trying to manually turn him. This is a procedure called external cephalic version (ECV) and is usually attempted when a woman is around 37–38 weeks pregnant. Your obstetrician will explain the exact procedure and any possible risks. It is said to be successful for around half of mothers (fewer for the women I see!) but not all babies and mothers are suitable candidates.

If your baby is still in the breech position at 38 weeks, it is very likely that your obstetrician will suggest you have an elective Caesarean section – probably a week later, when you are 39 weeks.

Oh no...not a Caesarean

For some, this news is fine – and to be completely rational, of course it's fine, and you don't have much choice. *All that matters is that you and your baby are OK – not the method of delivery.* And there are several pluses about knowing on exactly which date he will be born! But it's often hard to be rational, especially at the end of pregnancy. For many women, to be told they will need to have an elective Caesarean section is really upsetting news – especially if they are fit and healthy, and have been expecting and looking forward to a natural delivery. Even women who had psyched themselves up for birth rather than looking forward to it have arrived for a class to tell me with an expression of anguish, 'My baby's breech – I may have to have a Caesarean.'

Part of the reason the news is so upsetting for many women can again be blamed on the emotional changes that happen during pregnancy. Pregnant women like everything to be in order and find a sudden change of plan very difficult to cope with. It takes a week or two to adjust to things. And if a baby turns in the meantime, just as his mother is beginning to accept that she might need an elective Caesarean, she then comes into the next class and says (with an equal expression of anguish), 'Oh no, my baby's turned – I've got to have it naturally now.'

SIGNS OF IMMINENT LABOUR – BUT NO NEED TO GO IN!

Losing the Plug

This is a small lump of jelly that sits in the closed cervix as a barrier against any infection. At the end of pregnancy, if you are lucky, the Braxton Hicks contractions (see Chapter 6) will already be working on your closed cervix to soften and efface it in preparation for labour. If this is happening to you, it's possible you will go to the loo and find a lump of clear/whitish jelly – possibly streaked with watery blood. This is good news at the end of pregnancy because it means things are getting ready – but you don't have to go into hospital or phone your obstetrician or doctor, especially if it's two o'clock in the morning. Although you may well start contractions from any time, it is not unusual for women to lose their plug three weeks before going into labour.

What is more usual is for little bits of the plug to come away as the cervix 'softens'. At the end of pregnancy it is normal to have an increase in your pregnancy vaginal discharge, so the majority of women don't notice any bits of the mucous plug. If your membranes rupture, the amniotic fluid will wash it out.

Signs of Imminent Labour that You Realise only with Hindsight

Feeling Flu-like, Having Diarrhoea and Feeling or Being Sick

The evening before labour starts, many women will have what they might think of as a tummy upset – possibly a bout of diarrhoea and/or feeling sick. They will say, 'Oh dear, I think I've got a bug – I'm going to bed early. Let's hope I don't go into labour tonight.' And guess what? Interestingly enough, women who have really fast labours (six hours or so for their first baby) nearly always report back that they felt 'fluey' or rather unwell.

Hands and Knees!

This is another sign of early labour which you don't necessarily recognise at the time. It's fascinating how often women get on all fours during early labour (to help with the rotation of their baby's head in preparation for birth) and how they justify their possibly rather strange behaviour. I have taken second-time mothers for antenatal classes who have said the following: 'The night before I went into labour we went to a barbecue at my brother's house. I thought I was having contractions, but didn't want to make a fuss. Looking back, I can't believe that I let my niece sit piggy back on me while I crawled across the garden with her on my back.' Another: 'My husband is a banker and has an awful lot of shirts. The night before I went into labour, I spent a couple of hours on my hands and knees "colour-coding" all his shirts – it seemed quite a normal thing to do at the time.' And women will suddenly have a panic that the baby's room isn't clean enough or good enough and decide to paint the skirting boards. Or clean behind the cooker. I decided to hand-wash the sitting room carpet the evening before going into labour with my second child – totally out of character, but it seemed normal at the time.

WHEN WILL LABOUR START?!

At the very end of pregnancy, there may be quite a few false alarms. It is normal to wake up in the night with what feels like contractions and think: 'Is this it?' You will get up, make a cup of something and start to time them. More often than not, the contractions peter out and the woman goes back to bed – another interrupted night!

I'm a Week Overdue

This is probably another unforeseen scenario – everyone in your antenatal class has had their baby – you have been looking forward to a natural birth and, blow me down, you are now a week overdue. Not only are you pretty fed up but, worse still, at your last antenatal clinic the midwife mentioned induction, and you have heard that this is really 'unnatural'... Don't panic, everything will be OK and your baby will be worth waiting for.

Induction

The facts of the matter are: if your baby is two weeks overdue, he is much safer 'out' than 'in' (see page 99). And that is all that matters. There are other reasons, of course, for inducing a baby, such as your membranes having broken but you haven't spontaneously gone into labour, or if you develop pre-eclampsia (see page 48). If you are not sure why you are being offered an induction, ask your obstetrician or midwife – they will be able to explain. In spite of what people may tell you, babies are not induced because it is convenient for the obstetrician – quite simply, babies are induced because it is the safest option for the baby to be delivered.

How Do They Induce?

To a large extent, the method of inducing labour will depend on the condition of the woman's cervix:

Membrane Sweep

This is often the first suggestion if your cervix is effaced (see page 87). A sweep can be carried out by your GP, your midwife or your obstetrician. You are given a vaginal examination where the membranes are gently separated from the inner edge of the cervix, and this is an effective way of 'triggering' normal labour. Although many of you say it's not particularly comfortable, women don't report back that it's a painful procedure! And if you go into labour as a result of a sweep being performed at your doctor's surgery, you will have avoided having to go into hospital for the early stages.

Vaginal Pessary or Gel

If the cervix hasn't effaced, women are likely to be induced by a prostaglandin 'gel' or pessary, which is put straight into the vagina. Prostaglandins are produced naturally by your body, and at the end of pregnancy are responsible for 'softening' and shortening the cervix. The gel or pessary will be a synthetic form of this hormone (often 'Prostin'), which again should 'trigger' natural labour – the only difference being that you will spend all your labour in hospital, rather than the early stages at home. You are often asked to go into hospital in the evening, and given the gel or pessary, which will hopefully soften the cervix overnight. You are then given another dose in the morning, and possibly a further dose four hours later. But the individual responses to this are enormously variable – some women start contractions within a few hours and a few women don't respond at all.

Artificial Rupture of the Membranes (ARM)

If you have responded to the Prostin and your cervix has started to dilate, your midwife may rupture your membranes. Once the membranes have been broken, the body produces more prostaglandin, which will speed up labour. In fact, if you are admitted to hospital in labour and your membranes are still intact, it is likely your midwife will do an ARM in any case, for just this reason. The procedure involves another vaginal examination, during which the membranes are gently caught by a very small hook. This is not painful!

Intravenous Drip ('Syntocinon')

Syntocinon is a synthetic form of oxytocin – another natural hormone that makes the uterus contract. This type of induction means that the contractions are usually more frequent and powerful from the beginning – you miss out on the latent stage. Labour is more 'mechanised' in that your baby's heartbeat is always monitored, so you won't be able to move around. Because of this, it's sensible to ask for an epidural, if you want one, before the drip is set up. Syntocinon can also be used to accelerate or augment contractions once labour has started.

ORGANISING YOUR TIME WHEN YOUR BABY IS DUE ANY MINUTE

From 40 weeks, you have the problem of filling your time. Even if you have been booked in for an induction, most women describe the situation as 'living in a sort of void', and find it difficult to keep their spirits up! Well-meaning friends and family are ringing you constantly for 'any news?' For some reason this is incredibly irritating and makes you feel as though you have 'failed' to go into labour. You may want to keep your mobile off or on silent at the end of pregnancy, and change the message on your land line (but let your mother know that this is what you are doing!).

Try very hard to keep busy:

- Buy or borrow lots of books ('page turners' as well as the Russian classics you always promised yourself you would read when you had the time).
- Make sure you have somewhere to go (even if it's only for a facial or leg wax) or someone to meet every day.
- Fix something to do every evening – buy cinema tickets (you won't go again for a few months), and arrange for a good friend or two (whom you can cancel if necessary, so not a party) to come round for supper.
- Think positively – never again will you have the luxury of time completely to yourself...

Sooner or later you will have your baby – and he will be worth waiting for.

CHAPTER 11

how labour begins

This chapter looks at what you can expect to happen during the early stages of labour, and what you can do at home before going in to hospital.

SOMETHING'S HAPPENING AT LAST!

The start of regular contractions is by far the most usual beginning to labour. It may be that your Braxton Hicks contractions (see page 93) seem to be rather intrusive or just become increasingly regular. It may be that you have a dull backache or period-type pains – don't ignore these, even though they don't feel like proper contractions.

At this point, if you are booked in for an elective Caesarean section, you will need to go to hospital as soon as possible. Otherwise, for most of you there is no hurry – for the vast majority of first-time mothers, labour is a long process, and it takes two hours of regular contractions before ensuring that you are indeed in 'true' rather than 'false' labour. Most first-time mothers arrive at the hospital too early – when you go into labour you are generally expected to remain at home for a few hours, if you have had an uncomplicated pregnancy and you are more than 37 weeks pregnant. Hospitals don't want you rocking up as soon as you have your first contraction. In any case, you'll probably want to avoid the scenario of rushing into hospital to find your contractions have stopped and you are told you are not in labour and sent home again.

There are two exceptions to this:

1   **Get into hospital as quickly as possible if you are losing bright red blood.** If you are on your own, dial 999. If you are with someone else, and your own hospital is near, get them to drive you straight to the hospital you are booked into (ringing the labour ward on the way). The blood loss could result from a rare problem when a part of the placenta comes away from the uterine wall, which is a potential emergency. The hospital will be able to sort out where the blood is coming from and, if necessary, your baby will be delivered by an emergency Caesarean section.

2   **Ring your hospital if your waters have broken – regardless of whether or not you have any contractions.** Your baby is lying in amniotic fluid within a membrane, which in turn is contained by the uterus. Actually, the descriptive term 'waters gone' is misleading – it's not that the waters have 'gone' it's that the membrane has torn or split (spontaneous rupture of the membranes – SROM), allowing amniotic fluid to leak out.

In spite of popular belief, only a small percentage of labours (fewer than 10 per cent) start with the membranes rupturing – for many women their membranes rupture spontaneously a few hours into labour, and some will find that they don't rupture at all, and will be broken by the midwife when they are in labour (artificial rupture of the membranes – ARM).

How Do You Know for Sure that Your Waters Have 'Gone'?

Sometimes it's easy. You can lose amniotic fluid literally as a gush, in which case there isn't a problem realising what has happened, but for more it starts as a slight trickle or dampness.

There may be a gap between your baby's head and the cervix, so amniotic fluid will collect there, and it is then known as forewaters. If this is the case, there's usually no mistaking that your membranes have broken – you can lose up to a litre of fluid! This is probably something most pregnant women dread – quietly pushing a trolley round M&S when suddenly…but in all honesty this is very unlikely to happen, and if it does, rest assured that the relevant shop will be anxious to help you out and into hospital as soon as possible, probably with a free trolley of goodies. Funnily enough though, many women's membranes break at night or in the early morning as they get out of bed for yet another pee. And again, many women say that they actually hear what they describe as a 'pop' sound before amniotic fluid gushes over the mattress and the bedroom carpet. (And how pleased they were that they had put a bin liner under the mattress protector (see page 65)).

But if your baby is lying with his head right down on the cervix and the membranes then break, only a little fluid will be able to escape because the baby's head is in the way. If this is the case, you may find that you are damp, but not absolutely sure if it's amniotic fluid or perhaps leaking urine. At the end of pregnancy, however good your pelvic floor muscle may be, it is not uncommon to leak wee sometimes when you cough.

If you think your membranes might have broken but you are not sure, this is how to check:

1 Go to the loo and empty your bladder so there's no urine left to leak.
2 Tighten your pelvic floor muscles.
3 With your pelvic floor muscles still tightened, bear down as though you are trying to pee.

If you do leak fluid, it is likely to be amniotic fluid rather than wee. If you don't leak fluid, wait and see what happens over the next hour or so.

Once the membranes have broken, the amniotic fluid doesn't just drain away until there's none left. Clever nature continually replaces it – so it's a bit like the plug not fitting tightly in a bath of water, but the tap is dripping. This in turn means that if you are reasonably switched on, you will notice that you are damp through-out the day. If you are still not sure, it's probably best not to wear a sanitary towel (which will soak up the fluid) but just a pair of pants, which makes it easy for you to see if they are remaining dry. Amniotic fluid is colourless (unless the baby has passed meconium – see below) and has a distinctive and not unpleasant smell. It's quite difficult to describe smells – I would say it's a protein-like smell.

Having said that amniotic fluid is colourless, if you notice that you are losing fluid that is a brownish or greenish colour, you should get into hospital more quickly. While he is developing, a baby has a greenish/black substance in his gut called meconium, which he usually passes within 24 hours after birth. Sometimes he will open his bowels before or when you are in labour – and although he may be perfectly OK, it might also indicate that he is under stress, so this needs to be checked out at the hospital.

So Do I Have to Go to Hospital at this Point?

You might receive confusing advice. Even if you think your membranes have ruptured, some midwives will tell you to stay at home until you start contracting. But the obstetricians I have spoken to tell me that the safest advice is for women to go to hospital so it can be confirmed that their membranes have indeed ruptured and to monitor the baby's heart – even if they are then sent home again. There are two reasons for going in:

1 **It is important that the time the membranes break is recorded in your notes.** This is because once the membranes have broken, the uterus and your baby are unshielded from any bacteria that normally live happily in the vagina, putting you at risk from a bacterial infection if these bacteria decide to move upwards to pastures new, where they become less benign. As it happens, once the membranes have ruptured, hormone-like substances called prostaglandins are released which help 'trigger' and stimulate contractions, so most women go into labour spontaneously within 24 hours. (This is one of the reasons why your membranes, if still intact, may be artificially ruptured when you have been admitted to hospital in labour.) But sometimes this doesn't happen, and because of the risk of infection, these women will have their labour stimulated. This is why the time needs to be accurately recorded.

2 **There is an extremely rare chance of something called a cord prolapse (more likely if your baby is not engaged).** This is when the cord is lying next to or in front of the baby's head and loss of fluid allows the cord to slip down where it could be squashed during labour. The hospital can check for this rare problem simply by monitoring the baby's heart rate. If you are more than an hour's drive from the hospital you are booked into (such as staying with your parents) go to the nearest hospital and tell them your membranes have gone. The hospital will check that you don't have an infection and that your baby is fine. When you know all is well, you can then go home and phone the labour ward of your own hospital.

Once you have been checked over at your own maternity unit, it's quite usual to be sent home, especially if you haven't yet started contractions. So you will usually be sent home with instructions to take your temperature every four hours, and to return to the hospital around twelve hours later. If by the time you return to hospital you haven't spontaneously started labour, it is likely that you will be induced – simply to avoid the chance of infection.

REGULAR CONTRACTIONS

If you are in true labour, the contractions will become constant – each lasting about the same length of time with the gap in between also lasting the same length. They will continue for a period of two hours or more. One of the other ways of working out whether you are indeed in labour is to **go to bed and try and rest**. If you fall asleep, it is very unlikely you are in true labour! One of the things about the latent stage is that most women have a natural restlessness – they like to be able to get up, move around, sit down again and so on. This seems to make the contractions much less noticeable. Generally speaking, what women absolutely don't like in early labour is to be made to lie down – the contractions become more intrusive and they can't settle. So going to bed is a good idea – and if you don't fall into the usual group, and are in labour but do fall asleep – no harm done! Again the following has to be a generalisation – every woman is different, and you might not be Mrs Average in any way.

Early Labour while You Are Still at Home

Let's imagine that you are in the early stages of labour – you have had contractions most of the night, but you are coping with them well. You have phoned the hospital and been told to stay at home until the contractions are coming every 10 minutes. You will not be in a panic! This might be because you are just thoroughly sick of being pregnant, and at last something is happening; but contrary to what you might think in pregnancy, it is usual for women in early labour to find they have a sense of calm. So if you do find that you are anxious or uneasy, **ring your hospital and speak to a midwife**. If you want to, there is absolutely nothing wrong with asking if you can come in and be checked over.

You may or may not want your partner or anyone else with you – interestingly, many women prefer to be on their own! One woman said, 'Well, he was fine until he decided to cook himself a large fry-up to fortify himself for the labour. The smell was quite impossible for me to cope with.' But if you are happy for him to go into work, be sure that you tell him to keep his phone on, charged and with him!

What Should I Be Doing?!

Put away any expensive jewellery such as earrings and stoned rings, and take off your nail varnish. If by any chance you have to go to theatre, you will be asked to take off any stoned jewellery (as they may harbour bacteria). As one of my mothers said, 'I had to go to theatre for a Caesarean, so they told me to take off my earrings. I gave them to my husband who put them in his pocket, and it wasn't until we came home that he realised one of them was missing.' When you have checked that your labour bags are packed and ready to go (see page 159), this is the time to try out for real your breathing and relaxation (see page 95). You know the theory, and now you can start putting it into practice! Although you might find you can continue your normal breathing through a contraction at first, sooner or later, as they become stronger, you will notice you are beginning to want to hold your breath. So when the contraction starts you will sigh out and start your basic breathing.

Positions

Work out what position suits you best when you have a contraction – it is likely to be some sort of variation on leaning forwards. And on the whole, at the beginning of labour you will want to stay on your feet. Initially you will find that you may just lean forwards over the back of a sofa during a contraction. In fact, nearly all women use this position at some stage. Because you will instinctively want to tighten your muscles when you are leaning forward, it's sometimes helpful to 'hoola-hoop' your hips or move your pelvis up and down during a contraction. Alternatively, you might want to sit on a kitchen chair, facing the back and leaning against pillows.

It's worth trying a hands and knees position during a contraction, especially if you are getting backache. If you do this, put a pillow between your bottom and your heels as it's much more comfortable for you when you come up to sitting.

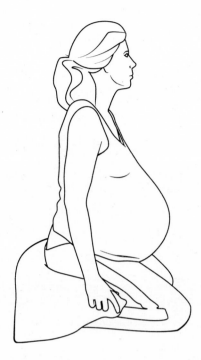

The important thing at this stage is to work out which positions work best for you during a contraction. The rule in labour is that **whatever position you can find that makes the pain easiest to cope with is the right position**. You don't have to look anything up in a reference book – just have the confidence to listen to your body. Your body will tell you what to do. I really mean it. And the advantage of being at home is that you can experiment and find out what works for you and what doesn't. As soon as you get into hospital you will lose confidence and find it much more difficult to trust your instincts – especially if you try a position such as getting on your hands and knees and find the pain is worse and you can't get up again without help!

Many women will want to get into a bath – and this is definitely worth a try. Apart from the fact that it whiles away some time, most women find lying in water soothing during contractions, and those women may go on to use a pool later in labour. But contrary to what you may read, water is not helpful for all women! Now is the best time to find out what is actually good for you. When you get to hospital it is likely that a midwife will suggest you get into a bath so it's helpful for you to find out in advance if this really does help you or not!

TENS (Transcutaneous Electrical Nerve Stimulation)

If you are going to use a TENS machine, now may be the time to ask someone to fit it on you. It is terribly important to regard this as something that will increase your pain tolerance as opposed to giving you relief from pain. A TENS machine will **not** give you a pain-free birth, but if you would like to have a 'natural' birth if possible, it might be worth considering.

TENS machines have been used for years by physiotherapists to help people with chronic pain, and about 20 years ago someone had the good idea of modifying one for women in labour. An obstetric TENS machine differs from those used for general purposes, so if you decide to hire one (such as from large branches of Boots) make sure it is the obstetric version.

It is a small hand-held unit with a battery inside. Attached to the unit are four wires ending in pads (electrodes). The electrodes are positioned in pairs onto your back with self-adhesive gel. One pair goes just below the shoulder blades and the second pair over the dimples in your pelvis at the bottom of your spine – the manual will show the precise places. When you turn the unit on, a mild electrical current (producing a tingling sensation) stimulates the nerve roots that supply the uterus – nowhere near the placenta or your baby. There are two types of current, which you change by a button attached to the machine:

1 **Continuous current** – used during a contraction (C for continuous – C for contraction!)

This current is supposed to 'scramble' and therefore reduce the pain messages to the brain produced by the contracting uterus.

2 **Pulsating current** – used between contractions

The body produces hormones called endorphins in response to pain – and when you have a high endorphin level, you experience a feeling of wellbeing. (You may recognise this feeling if you used to do gym workouts.) The pulsating current should give you just the same effect and is designed to boost your already high endorphin level.

Most women hire, rather than buy, a TENS machine and ask someone to put in on while they are at home. It needs to be fitted early in labour because it takes up to an hour for the electrical current to get the endorphin level up. Once the electrodes have been removed (perhaps to get into the bath or a pool) your endorphin level drops pretty quickly and it will take another hour with the TENS for it to rise again.

It's very difficult to know just how effective TENS machines are as there have been no satisfactory trials, but they are thought to increase a woman's pain threshold by between 10 and 20 per cent. We have taken several women for antenatal classes who used it for their first labour and said, 'I thought it wasn't working at all until I took it off, and then I realised it had been working really well.' Generally speaking, most mothers who used it in labour report that it was really helpful, and nearly all go on to use it again for their subsequent labours. But the important message is, even if you think it is useless, don't take it off until you have some other type of pain relief lined up.

Eating and Drinking

In the latent stage of labour you can eat and drink whatever you fancy – your body will tell you what you need. You should keep your energy and fluid levels up now, as it is unlikely that you will want to eat anything in the active stage.

When to Go to Hospital

At some stage you will decide that you want to go into hospital. Don't think you have to leave things as late as possible – if you find that you are on your hands and knees and don't want to get up – you are probably cutting things a bit fine! When you phone the labour ward, it is likely that the midwife will tell you not to come in until your contractions are ten minutes apart. This is a difficult one – during the latent stage, the frequency of contractions ranges from every five minutes apart to every twenty minutes apart – so understandably, midwives will take the mean, which is about every seven to ten minutes. But in fact it is the length and strength of the contractions themselves which is most relevant.

These are the general indications that you need to go in:

- Your contractions are regular and lasting 40 seconds or longer.
- You need to use your breathing.
- You want to go in.

The last point is quite important – you already know that most women go into hospital 'too early' with their first labour, but **women have a sixth sense which should always be taken seriously**. If you want to go to hospital – go. There is absolutely nothing wrong with getting in and having yourself and your baby checked over, even if you are sent home again.

When You Arrive at the Hospital

Admission procedures vary enormously, but at some stage you will have a vaginal examination to see how dilated you are. (You have to reach 10 cm dilation before you have the baby, but most women tend to arrive at the hospital when they are 3–4 cm dilated.) How dilated you are when you arrive at the hospital is pivotal information, as it will give you (and your partner) a general idea of how long a labour you are likely to be in for! If, for example, you have been in labour for two days and the midwife says, 'Great, Mrs Smith, you're 1 cm dilated,' you know you are going to be in for a longish labour! Conversely, you may have been in labour for only three hours, handling the contractions is not a problem but it is Friday evening and you are worried about the traffic, so you have gone in relatively early. You midwife may say (joy, oh joy) that you are already 6 cm dilated – you know you are going to be in for a shorter labour.

Monitoring Your Baby's Heartbeat

This is important because the monitoring will let the midwife know that your baby's cord is not being compressed during a contraction. But it may prove pretty uncomfortable for you because monitoring usually involves semi-sitting in bed with a tight belt round your tummy, which is attached by a wire to a screen at the side of the bed. This will show your baby's heartbeat and will give a printout of the contractions. For most women in labour, the last position they want to be in is leaning back in bed – you will realise the advantages of being upright and moving around! But try and put up with the awkward position if possible – the monitoring is not usually for more than 40 minutes, and as soon as everyone is happy that your baby is fine, you will be unhooked and allowed to move around again. If, however, you find it desperately uncomfortable, tell your midwife and she might be able to help you move into a different position, such as turning round to kneel up against the back of the bed, which will take the pressure off your bottom and still, hopefully, enable the monitor to stay in place.

The Antenatal and Labour Wards

One of the reasons for trying to arrive at the hospital when you are at the end of the latent stage is that most hospitals don't admit women to the labour ward until they are in the active stage of labour – which is when they are 3–4 cm dilated. So if you are admitted and still in the latent stage (or if by any chance the labour ward is full) you will probably go to a small antenatal ward where there are other women in early labour, accompanied by their partners.

This can sometimes be a bit grim – you may soon notice which of the other women in the ward with you went to antenatal classes and which didn't. You are not usually able to have an epidural on the antenatal ward, but gas and air should be available.

With any luck, though, you will be admitted quickly to the labour ward – usually a corridor with several separate side rooms – and here you are allocated your own midwife who will stay with you for the remaining length of her shift (eight hours). At this stage, you can breathe a sigh of relief – your midwife will help and advise you, and she will be your best friend for the next few hours! By now you will probably be in the active stage and can continue with your breathing, possibly decide that you would like to use the birthing pool if it's available, or alternatively you might want some pain relief…

CHAPTER 12

labour continues...
and possible pain releif

The active stage of labour is when you may start to need some (or more) pain relief. In this chapter we look at the options available to you, and their pros and cons.

CONTINUING WITH YOUR BREATHING

The point of doing some breathing and relaxation through contractions is to help you conserve energy. It has to be said that the breathing won't make the pain disappear, although it will make the contractions more manageable. All you have to do is see how things go – you are not expected to do some ghastly assault course; you are just hoping to breathe through the contractions for as long as is reasonable (for you) as opposed to as long as is humanly possible!

It is important to think of each contraction in a positive way – a step nearer to your baby. As soon as the contraction starts, think 'Good' (rather than 'Oh God, not another one'), sigh out, lean forwards, relax the muscles you have control over, and start your basic breathing (see page 96). Relaxing your muscles may just mean pulling your shoulders down towards the floor (to prevent them being glued to your ears) and making sure your hands are not tightly fisted.

As the contractions become more powerful, you will notice that your breathing automatically becomes quicker and you just can't keep to your basic breathing. Powerful contractions will not allow you to breathe slowly – the more powerful the contraction, the quicker your breathing will become. (This is why it's so difficult to practise breathing during antenatal classes – you tend to feel dizzy because you are altering your respiration rate without the need to do so.) At some point, you will notice that your breathing is too rapid to keep to nose/mouth breathing and you will have to mouth-breathe only. The fastest breathing you can possibly do is very light panting. What you are aiming to do is keep your breathing as slow as possible for as long as possible – so you have always got some-where to 'take' your breathing.

The rate of your breathing at the peak of each contraction will give you an idea about how well you are coping. If your contrac-tions are lasting for 60 seconds, and 30 seconds into the contraction you have to transfer to mouth breathing – you are clearly doing fine. If, however, 20 seconds into a 60-second contraction, you haven't reached the peak and you are already panting – things are not fine. The contraction hasn't reached its peak and you can't breathe any more quickly. Help! A few contractions like this might mean you may want to think about pain relief.

Your midwife will give you an internal examination every four hours. Some of you will find that you are coping pretty happily with your contractions and you are dilating at a rate of around a centimetre an hour – all good! Some of you will find that although you are dilating well, you are absolutely exhausted, and need some pain relief in order to recharge your batteries. And some of you will simply feel you have had enough pain and would like a break…

THINKING ABOUT PAIN RELIEF

As usual, the most relevant factors in all this are the length of your labour and the position that your baby is in. From the women I have seen, I don't believe that some women have a 'low pain threshold' – and it's certainly not helpful to be told this when you are in labour. Pain threshold is very dependent on the length of time you have been in labour – missing out on two nights' sleep automatically lowers anyone's pain threshold.

When it comes to pain relief, the figures I have gathered from the women I have taught at antenatal classes are quite interesting: 80 per cent of our first-time mothers have an epidural, but 80 per cent of second- or third-time mothers have 'natural' childbirth, using only gas and air. These are the same women – but subsequent labours are nearly always quicker, so the mother is much less tired. So, I conclude that most first-time mothers need pain relief not necessarily because they are in dire agony, but because they are knackered and need a break, and having some sort of pain relief means they will be in a fit state to push their baby into the world.

No mother should be made to have 'natural' childbirth by default. By that I mean pain relief is withheld from her until it's 'too late' because the person looking after her believes it's 'better' for a mother not to have pain relief, even if she wants it. It isn't anyone else's decision but yours! It really doesn't matter long-term whether you had an epidural or a 'natural' birth – honestly. Natural childbirth doesn't go on your CV, and frankly, even if it did, no-one would care!

So How Will I Know What to Ask for?

There are three different choices of pain relief generally available, and which you opt for depends on how dilated you are at the time. Here is a rough guide:

- Pethidine: Latent stage, before 3–4 cm dilation.
- Epidural: Beginning of the active stage, 3–4 cm to 7–8 cm dilation.
- Gas and Air (Entonox): 8 cm onwards (or while waiting for an epidural).

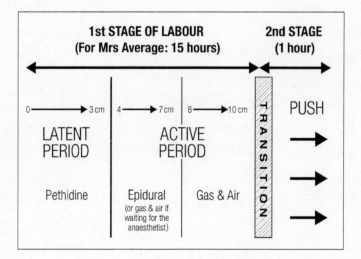

Pethidine

This is a pain-relieving drug which is given as an intramuscular injection by your midwife. It will kick in within 20 minutes and last between two and four hours. It is most useful in early labour if exhaustion is more of a problem than the pain and it is too soon to have an epidural. The effects will make you feel sleepy and slightly disorientated, but at the same time 'removed' from the pain – women describe it as 'the pain was displaced to the other side of the room' or 'the pain seemed to be hanging off the end of the bed'. You won't be able to walk around because you will be a bit woozy.

The downsides to pethidine are:

- It makes most people feel sick – so you may be given an anti-sickness drug (anti-emetic) at the same time.
- If you find you don't like the effects of feeling 'out of it', you're stuck with them until the drug wears off.
- It crosses the placenta, so if your baby is born within three hours or so of you having been given pethidine, he will be a little drowsy as well. (That's one of the reasons for suggesting you don't have it after 3–4 cm dilation.)

As it happens, very few of the mothers I see use pethidine, but on some occasions it is incredibly helpful. For instance, if you have been up pacing around your house without any sleep (because the contractions stop you sleeping) for two nights and arrive at the hospital exhausted and tearful to be told 'You're 1 cm dilated' – pethidine would be the choice to go for. Irrational as it might be (but no-one in labour is rational) you think, 'Oh my God, I've been in labour for 48 hours and I can't even dilate beyond 1 cm. What on

193

earth am I going to do? What on earth is going to happen?' You will probably be told you are too early on in labour to be given an epidural, but you desperately need to be able to relax and to get some sleep. Interestingly enough, contrary to what one would expect (because you go to bed, rather than walk around) women in this situation often have an hour's sleep and wake up to find they're now 3 cm dilated. And refreshed – and therefore calmer and feeling more in control.

Epidurals

This is a local anaesthetic, which completely removes the pain (for nearly everyone). The enormous advantage of epidurals is that they don't affect you systemically – this means that your brain is as lucid as ever! The best time for an epidural is when you are between 3 cm and 8 cm dilated – you can't *not* have an epidural afterwards but 'eight is a bit late' (see below).

An anaesthetist has to be called to set it up. It is important to bear in mind that anaesthetists on a labour ward may have a number of women who need their help, or they may be in theatre looking after a woman having a Caesarean. This means that you won't be able to bank on the anaesthetist arriving within minutes of you asking for one. He can take up to an hour to arrive – not because he doesn't care, but because he is tied up with someone else.

Because of this, you need to consider the possibility of requesting an epidural earlier rather than later – you don't want to leave things until you are absolutely desperate. (It's unlikely that your midwife will suggest that you have an epidural without you requesting one first.) But you can always use gas and air (see page 198) to tide you over once you know the anaesthetist is coming.

So What Happens?

The anaesthetist will ask you to lie on your side on the bed with your knees pulled up to your chest, or sometimes sit on the side of the bed leaning forwards (this alone can prove to be tricky when you are nine months pregnant). This is so he can feel the bones more easily at the lower end of your spine in order to find the correct land-mark for the injection. He gives you a local anaesthetic – a pinprick under the skin – and this is likely to be the only thing you find uncomfortable. You will feel pressure on your back as he glides a fine needle between two lumbar (lower) vertebrae, and into what is called the epidural space.

All this is done *between* your contractions, so you don't have to worry about trying to keep still during a contraction. And this is the reason why 3–7 cm dilation is the best time – at this stage the gap between your contractions is between three and five minutes, so with any luck the anaesthetist has a clear five minutes at a time to site the epidural. Once you get beyond 7 cm, the gap between contrac-tions closes to two-and-a-half to three minutes so he has less time to get it in position, so by the time the epidural is set up you may be fully dilated and may not want it to start to take effect just at the point you are ready to push.

Once the epidural needle is in place, all is nearly done. The local anaesthetic is delivered via the needle – this does not pass over to your baby – and very quickly you will have no pain from the tummy button downwards. A miracle! Anaesthetists are so wonderful! A tiny tube (catheter) is then threaded through the needle, the needle taken out (so you are *not* left with a needle sticking out of your back) and the part of the catheter remaining outside is plastered to your lower back and then up to your shoulder so your midwife can top up the anaesthetic when you ask for it.

Within the last 10 years or so, there has been a radical development in epidurals. The anaesthetic previously used affected the nerves that supply the leg muscles as well as the nerves that register pain. The epidurals used now are a combination of analgesics that cleverly block only the sensory (pain) nerves, but not the motor nerves that supply your muscles. This means that you can move your legs (and even walk around) rather than feeling as though they are encased in a concrete boot. These epidurals are called 'mobile' or 'walking' epidurals, or sometimes 'low-dosage' epidurals, and are now nearly always used in large hospitals. The term 'low-dosage' is an understandably worrying description – but it doesn't mean only a small amount of epidural. You should still experience complete pain relief.

Downsides

An epidural will lower a woman's blood pressure. (In some cases, if a woman in labour has high blood pressure, her obstetrician may suggest that she has an epidural solely to lower her blood pressure.) To compensate, most women are given a litre of fluid, via an intravenous drip in the back of their hand, which keeps their blood volume stable – this will take around 40 minutes to be absorbed. During this time, the baby will be monitored in the same way as when you were first admitted to hospital. Once the fluid has been absorbed, for the vast majority of you, the drip comes down and the monitor comes off. But of course a litre of fluid will mean that your bladder has filled, so you will need to empty it. (A full bladder will stop your baby's head moving through your pelvis.) With a mobile epidural, peeing is relatively straightforward – you can pad off to the loo, and with any luck there won't be a problem. When you get back to your bed, you may want to lean forward against it while you rotate your hips (see page 182), but most of you will climb back in and get some rest at last. If you find that you can't empty your bladder, your midwife will empty it by passing a small catheter into your bladder – a frightening idea, but completely painless.

An irritating problem for quite a few women is that an epidural will slow down their contractions, which in turn slows down their labour. This is a good reason to wait and ask for an epidural when (and if) you need one, rather than at the onset of the first contraction. And if you are thinking: 'Do I need an epidural? Actually I'm not sure I fancy the drip' – you probably don't need one! If the contractions become less effective, you may be given Syntocinon (see page 172) to accelerate them and avoid a protracted labour. This is administered (and at the same time the amount carefully monitored) via the drip in the back of your hand. All women who are given Syntocinon must have their baby's heart monitored at the same time, so you won't be able to move around, and will find yourself in a much more mechanised and medically managed labour. And women who have an epidural have a slightly increased chance of needing an assisted delivery (forceps or ventouse, see page 210).

Dural Tap

Statistically it's safer to have an epidural than to have a baby. Very, very occasionally, there is a problem in that the epidural needle 'nicks' the membrane that surrounds the spinal cord (dura), and this is called a dural tap. This does *not* cause permanent paralysis, but can give you a bad headache when you sit up. The anaesthetist will know if this has happened, and in a very few cases you may have your baby delivered by forceps. After delivery, the 'nick' can be sealed fairly easily by a procedure called a 'blood patch', which involves taking a small amount of blood from a vein in the arm and injecting it into the epidural site.

Many women complain of lower back pain after childbirth. If they have had an epidural, it is understandable to assume it is the result of this. Actually, there isn't any link between long-term lower back pain and epidurals.

When I talk to women about their labour, everyone who has had an epidural tells me how wonderful they are. The descriptions range from 'the best thing in the word' to 'bliss'. One particular woman said: 'It's like dying and going to heaven.' Nobody has ever told me that they wished they hadn't had one.

Gas and Air (Entonox)

This is a quick-acting pain-relieving agent (nitrous oxide and oxygen) which is self-administered via a mask or mouthpiece that you hold yourself. It doesn't cross the placenta. It is an ideal method of short-term pain relief at the end of the first stage of labour (after 8 cm dilation), as it is best not to use it for more than a three-hour period. Inexplicably, a birth where the woman has only gas and air is called a 'natural' birth.

The gas and air will do two things – suppress the pain (considerably) and at the same time give you a 'high' or 'buzz'. Unlike pethidine, it only gives you the effect while you are breathing it into your system – once you take away the mask or mouthpiece, you breathe the Entonox out of your body, so you are back to normal. The idea is for you to use it *during* contractions and let it wear off between contractions. But as there is a latency period of around 10–

20 seconds (depending on how deeply you breathe) between breathing the gas and you noticing the effects, this timing is very important. In fact, most women who say that gas and air didn't 'work' will have got the timing wrong.

The way to use it is to start breathing the mixture into your lungs *as soon as* the contraction starts, so you have time to get the maximum amount of gas and air into your body. Then when you are halfway through the contraction plus 10 seconds, you take the mask/mouthpiece away, so the effects have worn off by the end of the contraction and you are gas and air-free between contractions. You will need to time the contractions so you know how long they are lasting. Your partner is usually a great help with this timing – he can time the contraction and tell you when to take the mask off (but not snatch it away from you, which you will find irritating).

Timing of gas and air

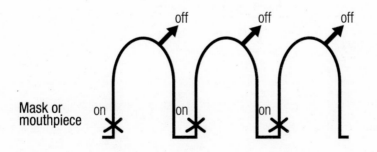

After about three hours the body accommodates to and becomes 'saturated' with Entonox. Nothing disastrous happens, but it means you won't come down very well between the contractions and are likely to feel uncomfortably spaced out and confused all the time – not a good feeling for you and it makes it difficult for you to follow your midwife's instructions. But when you are 8 cm dilated, bearing in mind most women dilate a centimetre an hour, you shouldn't need to use it for more than three hours before being ready to push. Although you wouldn't start to use gas and air at 4 cm and hope it will see you through the rest of labour, it is also a very good 'crisis' drug, such as:

- when you are waiting for the anaesthetist to arrive with the epidural
- during internal examinations
- when you want to push and your midwife is saying 'not yet'
- if the sensation of your baby's head crowning is unpleasant

Downsides
As with pethidine, gas and air makes some women feel nauseated, and some don't like the feeling of light-headedness.

THE END OF THE FIRST STAGE OF LABOUR (TRANSITION)

Transition is the very last half centimetre of dilation before the cervix is ready for you to push – the transition between the first and second (pushing) stage of labour itself. If you are having your baby privately, this is the time your obstetrician is likely to arrive.

For some, this last 20 minutes of the first stage is really tough. Three changes may happen:

1 **The contractions seem to lose their rhythm.** They may feel as though they reach their peak, start to abate but then seem to peak again. Women will say, 'I don't know when the contraction is starting – I seem to have a contraction all the time.' It's almost as if the uterus is not sure whether it is contracting in order to dilate the cervix or contracting in order to push the baby out.

2 **Physical changes.** These may include feeling sick, being sick (not great) and sometimes apparently histrionic shivering (which can be very frightening for your partner).

3 **Emotional changes.** You may think to yourself, 'I've absolutely had enough. I think I'm going to die and no-one cares. I'm *never* having a baby again.' I always ask second-time mothers if they experienced any transition changes, and they have told wonderful stories. Many have reported back that they have said, 'Right, that's it, I'm not having the baby today, I'm going home.' Some have started to get out of bed (drip in tow) and headed off for the hospital lift, regardless of the midwife and husband's physical restraints. Some women may swear at whoever is attending them – often using swear words that are totally out of character for them outside their home. One second-time mother told the class, 'I said to my husband – actually you've been a total disappointment ever since I married you.' I'm not making any of the above up! It is rather important that your partner is aware that these emotional changes are possible – if he thinks he's in for a sentimental togetherness with the arrival of your first baby and you hit a tricky transition, he'll have a bit of a shock.

Having said all this, most women will reach 10 cm and have a strong urge to push with none of the above...

CHAPTER 13

second stage – the actual birth

VAGINAL DELIVERY

When your cervix is fully dilated (10 cm) you are ready to push your baby into the world. In fact, if you haven't had an epidural, you probably won't need to be told that you've reached this stage because for most women the urge to bear down or push at this point is so powerful it's almost involuntary – you can hardly stop yourself. At the same time, many women feel they urgently and desperately need to open their bowels. They almost certainly won't and don't, but the pressure of the baby's head squashing the lower bowel produces the same sensation.

Your midwife will (and must) examine you before you start to push, just to check that the cervix has completely pulled back over the baby's head. Occasionally, a part of the cervix becomes trapped between the baby's head and the pubic bone of the mother's pelvis. This is called an anterior lip – it happens to about 1 in 10 mothers and is a real nuisance! If this is the case, your midwife will ask you not to push until the contractions have freed this last bit of the cervix – which is not the instruction you want to hear if your urge to push is overwhelming. If you have real trouble stopping yourself bearing down, it's worth trying the following:

- Getting on your hands and knees with your head down and your bottom in the air – usually this position reduces your urge to push.
- Doing 'huff-puff' breathing you hopefully learnt in antenatal classes – if not, your midwife will show you. This is repeated light 'blowing out a candle' breathing, which stops you holding your breath and pushing down.
- Using Entonox (see page 198).

If you have had an epidural, you won't have a strong urge to push so an anterior lip will be less of a problem for you.

Provided your baby's heartbeat is steady, some midwives might suggest you wait for a bit before starting to push if your baby is still relatively high in your pelvis or because you have decided to let your epidural wear off a little. With an epidural still working, you won't feel a strong urge to bear down, but even so, it is perfectly possible to push out your baby. But the decision as to whether to let the epidural wear off for the second stage is completely up to you – you may well decide to have it topped up. Much will depend on how you feel at the time, how long you have had the epidural in, and the position of your baby. You don't need to make up your mind as to what to do about your epidural until you are actually ready to push.

What Position Will I Be in?

In your antenatal classes you may discuss and practise all sorts of different positions in which to give birth. Squatting, kneeling up against the back of the bed, kneeling on all fours, lying on your side or sitting upright on the bed are most of the options. But it's really difficult to know what position will be right for you until it comes to the time – everything (as usual) is so dependent on the position of your baby, how long you have been in labour, what your midwife or obstetrician suggests and what feels right for you when you start to push. Just see how you feel at the time! If you have spent the end of your labour on your hands and knees, you may want to remain in this position when you deliver your baby. If you have been propped up on the bed, you may find you are happy to remain in bed but supported by more pillows. The only position you are most unlikely to find helpful is lying flat on your back – this will mean that you won't have gravity to help you and will feel that you are literally pushing your baby uphill.

For many of you, when you are ready to start pushing, the back support of your bed can be usefully moved forward so you are in a semi-sitting position with your legs separated and bent at the knee. Sometimes you might find it helpful to have a midwife and possibly your partner supporting each leg for you during a contraction. For most women this feels OK and works perfectly well. The important thing is to listen in to your body and if the position you start off in doesn't feel right, tell your midwife (and your partner) and she will suggest different positions and help you find one that is better for you.

Pushing Your Baby Out

During the second stage, your task is to help the uterus push your baby out into the world. You need to work with your contractions, which by now will be coming every two to four minutes and lasting between 60 and 90 seconds. This feels very strange, even if you've already had five babies! Your midwife will keep saying to you, 'Push into your bottom, push into your bottom,' which is exactly what you need to do. It will help if you think of your diaphragm (the horizontal muscle that runs under your ribcage) as the plunger in a cafetière-type of coffee maker, and initiate the downward pushing movement from there. Many women say the nearest analogy is simply to imagine that you are extremely constipated and having to pass a melon. At the same time, it will help enormously if you *relax your pelvic floor muscles*, and this will be easiest if you keep your mouth and jaw muscles relaxed. (This sounds a little odd, but it's true!) If you are in a sitting position, it will also help if you try and 'aim' your baby towards the end of the bed. Some women find it helpful to imagine they are giving birth to a Wellington boot – toe first. The toe of the boot (your baby's head) has to point downwards in order to duck under your pelvic bone in front, and then goes back upwards to its normal position in order to be born.

When women tell me about their delivery, nearly everyone says, 'I had no idea I was going to have to push so hard.' For most women, this bit is really hard work – especially if it's your first baby. But, interestingly, many women say that unlike the pain of the contractions during the first stage of labour, the pain during the second stage was not too much of a problem. The uncomfortable bit is the stretching sensation – but of course, your baby is nearly there. You may want your partner to mop your brow or give you ice to suck while you take the time between contractions to recharge your batteries. What is most important is that when the next contraction starts, he helps you get back into the right position for you. If you are sitting, it's usual to slip downwards whilst you are pushing, and he will need to give you a hand sitting up again.

When your baby's head is pushing against your pelvic floor muscles it produces a really strange sensation. Because the muscles, and the nerves that supply them, are very stretched, you will probably find it impossible to differentiate between your anus and your vagina. It's quite normal to have a moment's panic that your baby is going to be born through your bottom rather than the conventional exit. This isn't going to happen!

As your baby's head starts to emerge, there will be a couple of contractions when you feel that nothing can stretch any further. Trust your midwife or obstetrician, and listen carefully to what she or he tells you to do. Push only when you are told to do so. When your baby's head is born, your midwife will put her hand on his head and say to you, 'Stop pushing – pant.' This is because she needs to check that the cord is not round his neck (this is not uncommon) and, if it is, to gently loop it over his head with her fingers, before he is delivered. Once the cord has been checked, one or two more small pushes and the baby rotates again so that his shoulders are delivered. And suddenly…there he is.

Many of you will read the above paragraphs and think that all this might be rather embarrassing. It won't be. It is an enormous privilege to be present when a woman gives birth – ask any professional and they will tell you that however many births they have attended, each one is always exciting and moving. In fact, I would say that although it's really good having a baby yourself, being allowed to watch someone else have a baby is much better – in fact, it's fantastic.

And Finally – the Placenta

A few minutes later, you will notice some more contractions as your uterus starts to expel the placenta, which has now done its job. Generally, this stage is a non-event as far as you are concerned, but there are potentially serious problems if this bit doesn't go smoothly (a post-partum haemorrhage or retained placenta). Most hospitals automatically give women an injection of a drug called Syntometrine, which is designed to prevent the above complications. Occasionally, some hospitals will ask you whether or not you want this drug – I can't think of a good reason to refuse it and I have known it to save lives.

Stitches

When the placenta is safely away (it looks like a large lump of liver) you are likely to need some stitches. The majority (about 70 per cent) of women will have a small tear in their skin and pelvic floor muscles. Although it sounds horrific, don't be frightened because you probably won't notice. Some women will need an episiotomy (a cut under local anaesthetic) to prevent serious tearing extending to the anal sphincter muscle. You probably won't know what has needed to be done – and it doesn't matter long-term whether you've had a small natural tear or an episiotomy. Trust your midwife or obstetrician to do what she feels is the best for you.

If your tear needs to be stitched, or you have had an episiotomy which always needs to be stitched, your legs will be placed up in stirrups (lithotomy position) so that whoever is stitching can see exactly what she or he is doing. You should not feel any pain at all. If you have had an epidural, it will be topped up for this, and if you haven't, you will be given a local anaesthetic. It takes a few minutes to start working, but if it is not enough you *must* tell whoever is stitching you. They can't read your mind! There's something odd about women who have just given birth – they are so incredibly grateful to whoever has delivered their baby, they worry that they may be causing trouble or being a bit of a wimp if they 'complain' that it hurts when they are being stitched up afterwards. This is clearly nonsense, but a very good example of how vulnerable a newly delivered mother can be.

All the above usually takes an hour or so – but sometimes things don't progress as quickly or as smoothly as your midwife would like, and medical input may be required.

When an Obstetrician Might Be Called... (by Lorin Lakasing)

In many countries routine antenatal care is provided by obstetricians. In the UK, we have a shortage of obstetricians but we are lucky enough to have midwives. Thus most women never see an obstetrician throughout their pregnancy and delivery unless they develop complications. But fear not! If you do meet an obstetrician along the way, it is not always bad news. Most of the time the midwife simply wants a bit of reassurance or support, and this should not be taken as a sign that things are going wrong. Of course, the type of doctor a pregnant woman is most likely to meet is not an obstetrician but an anaesthetist for insertion of an epidural. However, there are a few clinical situations in which an obstetrician might be involved and they are outlined below. I have concentrated on these, not necessarily because they are common, but because they can cause concern.

Assisted Delivery

Labour is exhausting and the pushing part in particular is hard work. Occasionally either mother or baby just run out of steam at this point and you may need assistance in the form of an instrumental delivery. This procedure is carried out by an obstetrician and usually performed in your delivery room, although occasionally you may be transferred to an operating theatre. There are many different types of instruments that are used in this situation but, broadly speaking, they fall into two main categories:

- the ventouse cup (a suction cup that is applied to the crown of baby's head)
- forceps (these look like salad servers and lock in the middle so that they cradle the baby's head)

Both sound fairly unattractive but do not worry. Some 15 per cent of babies are born this way and complications are very, very, very rare. After a ventouse delivery, your baby will have a small bruise on the crown of the head, and after a forceps delivery you might see some compression marks by the side of baby's cheeks. These all disappear within two to three days and have no long-term consequences.

Perineal Tears

The vast majority of first-time mothers who deliver vaginally will sustain a perineal tear. Not really a surprising statement if you think of the parameters involved! Most of these tears are very small and require just a few stitches. You will be a bit sore for a few days but there are usually no long-term consequences. Very rarely, some women are unfortunate enough to sustain very large or deep tears which can affect the anal sphincter (the ring of muscle that is responsible for maintaining bowel continence), and the prospect of having one of these third-degree tears, as they are called, quite understandably terrifies many women. Try not to be worried. Firstly, it is very rare, and secondly, if it is recognised and dealt with immediately after delivery it is very unlikely that you will have any long-term symptoms. Your obstetrician will use special techniques to sew you back together again, and women who are unlucky enough to have had such a tear or who suffer symptoms long after delivery will usually be followed up at a specialist clinic where a comprehensive assessment of the pelvic floor muscles is undertaken and appropriate help given.

CAESAREAN DELIVERY – LOWER SEGMENT CAESAREAN SECTION (LSCS)

It's important that you read this bit! (See also page 99.) Problems occasionally arise during labour that necessitate a fit and healthy woman having an unexpected Caesarean. No hospital makes the decision to give a woman in labour a Caesarean for any other reason than that her, or her baby's, life is at risk. So, thank goodness for Caesareans!

So What Happens?

Generally speaking, if you are having a Caesarean with an epidural, your partner will go with you. (You will appreciate him being there – in spite of him looking strangely unfamiliar wearing a gown and a hat!) At some point some of your pubic hair will be shaved, as the incision is made just below the hair line, and this area needs to be as sterile as possible. An anaesthetist will check that your epidural is topped up to a high enough level for you to feel no pain during the operation. This means you won't be able to move your legs, which feels rather odd.

You will lie on a bed and the staff will fix a screen below your chest so you cannot see anything. Your husband will sit one side of you and either an anaesthetist or a midwife will sit on the other side – so you have two people to talk to. It takes about 10 minutes to deliver your baby and you really won't feel any pain. Some women describe a slight 'tugging' sensation – one woman described her Caesarean as 'a bit like someone else rummaging around in your handbag'! As soon as your baby is born he is passed over the screen for you to hold. Magic! You will probably pass him to your husband pretty quickly while the placenta is delivered and you are stitched up. This takes longer than getting the baby delivered.

Immediately after the Operation...

You will rest in the recovery room for an hour or so before going down to the postnatal ward. During this time, your baby will be with you, and as your epidural wears off, the staff will give you more pain relief, take your blood pressure and generally check that all is OK. Don't be surprised to find you have an alarming number of small tubes attached to you:

- A drip attached to the back of your hand. This is usually taken down after an hour or so.
- A catheter draining urine from your bladder to a bag attached to the side of the bed. **Do not panic** – this will be taken out within 24 hours. (Meanwhile it's very handy as you don't have to get up and go to the loo!)

- Possibly a tube draining fluid from your abdomen – again into a bag attached to the bed. This will also be removed within 24 hours.

This time following a Caesarean birth is just as wonderful for you and your partner as it would be if you had a vaginal delivery.

YOUR BABY

At the moment of birth, whoever is looking after you generally becomes quite silent. This doesn't mean anything has gone wrong; it is because everyone is concentrating hard on your baby to make sure everything continues to go well. Although some babies will take their first breath as their head appears, others won't start to breathe on their own for up to a minute. And although it's wonderfully reassuring for everyone to hear a lusty cry, some babies don't cry immediately (or even at all) and are still perfectly OK.

When your midwife delivers your baby she will probably put him onto your tummy before she clamps the umbilical cord (with what look like two small freezer-food clips) and cuts it between the clips. This doesn't hurt your baby. Or perhaps she may ask your husband if he wants to cut the cord – and he may or may not want to. You may be given your baby to hold at this point, but if you don't want to hold your baby before he has been checked over and wrapped, say so. The same applies if you don't want your baby delivered onto your tummy. Everyone is different – there isn't a 'right' or a 'wrong' thing to do, and you don't have to do anything you don't feel comfortable about.

Your baby is then checked over (see below) on a little table near your bed with a warming lamp over it – babies lose heat very quickly. He will be fitted with an identification bracelet and wrapped in a swaddling sheet or blanket before being given to you. Some women find that immediately after birth, they start to shake uncontrollably – so much so that they are nervous about their ability to hold their baby safely. Don't panic if this happens to you. The shaking will stop and in the meantime let your husband hold your baby so you can look at him (or both of them!).

The Apgar Score

This is a way in which professionals can quickly check that your baby is in good shape and not needing special attention. It is taken as soon as possible after birth and repeated at five minutes. The score out of 10 is based on the following five observations:

- heart rate
- colour
- breathing
- muscle tone
- reflex response

Don't worry if your baby doesn't score a perfect 10 immediately – only a few do – but most will score between 8 and 10 at five minutes after birth. Babies that need an emergency Caesarean section may score slightly lower than babies who have a very straightforward birth.

Your Baby's Appearance

For most of you who haven't seen a newly born baby before, some things about him might be alarming:

- Before your baby starts to breathe on his own you might be worried that he looks a bluish colour and perhaps a bit lifeless. In fact, even when they breathe on their own, new babies remain quite blotchy for a little time.

- The shape of his head can look a little weird. There are five individual skull bones, and when a baby is born they are designed to move a little so they can 'mould' in order to fit through the mother's pelvis. It is usual and normal for a newborn baby's head to look asymmetrical and this will disappear over the next 24 hours or so. The moulding does not affect his brain and doesn't require the emergency attentions of a cranial osteopath.

- He will be wet – because he has been bathed in amniotic fluid.

- He may have some white creamy substance (vernix) over his body.

- He can have fine downy hair over his chest and even forehead (this can be a bit of a shock, as you might privately think he looks a little like a monkey).

- Boy babies have very large testicles in relation to their penis.

- Girl babies may have swollen labia or slightly enlarged breasts.

- There may be some blood on him – if there is, it will be yours, not his.

- If he has had an assisted delivery, there may be some bruise marks on his cheek from a forceps delivery or a swelling on the back of his head from a ventouse delivery. These will disappear.

TIDYING YOU UP

Hopefully, your midwife will have time to help you wash and change into a fresh nightdress. Do not be alarmed if you find that you already need a new sanitary pad – you will be losing blood from where the placenta was attached to the uterus, and for most women, this blood loss (called lochia) is rather heavier than expected. In fact, some women will find they need to wear two sanitary pads overlapping. If your stitches are hurting at this stage, ask for some painkillers – a painful bottom is not going to help you fall in love with your baby or help your breasts release colostrum.

If she hasn't already done so, your midwife will help you put your baby to your breast. Babies have a strong suckling reflex in the first hour after birth, and their sucking will help 'kick-start' lactation. But putting your baby to your breast for the first time ever can be a tricky business, and at this stage for most mothers doesn't necessarily feel particularly 'natural'. It's reassuring to have the experience and support of the midwife who has just delivered you, particularly if your baby decides not to suckle.

THE THREE OF YOU

Hospitals recognise the need for new parents to have some time on their own, but things depend very much on how busy they are. Ideally, you will be left alone for an hour, with a desperately needed cup of tea (and anything it's possible to eat), before being transferred to the postnatal ward. Unless you are vomiting, which is not unusual although I don't know why, this time is magic – your baby is likely to be lying quietly in your arms or in his crib, just looking around or asleep.

Although at this stage it is quite normal for women to feel depersonalised or just plain exhausted, with any luck you will feel on an amazing 'high', as though you are the only person in the world who has managed to give birth to a baby. As indeed, you now have.

THE POSTNATAL WARD

You will be transferred to the postnatal ward – maybe for six hours or perhaps for three days. If you are an NHS patient in London, you may be a little alarmed to find that there seem to be very few midwives, and those who are around are all very busy. You will still need the help of your partner – don't let him leave you until you have enough pain relief and easy access to fresh sanitary pads.

If You Have Had a Caesarean Section

You still lose blood (lochia) in exactly the same way as you would after a vaginal delivery. You will find that it hurts to cough, sneeze or laugh – if you support your stitches with a folded sanitary pad, this will help.

If you are in pain, tell the staff. I would suggest you take every painkiller on offer because when you are in pain, you are not able to move around, and this will slow down your recovery and spoil the enjoyment of your beautiful baby. Pain won't help with breastfeeding either. Although painkillers do pass through your milk, no hospital will give you anything that will harm your baby – and that's why you need to take what your obstetrician or doctor prescribes rather than buying something over the counter. Before you go home, make sure you are given an adequate supply of painkillers.

Don't be afraid to ask a midwife to lift your baby in and out of his cot – you may find it frightening to do this on your own for a day or two. If there doesn't seem to be anyone around to help you, ask another mother.

You will probably stay in hospital for two or three nights. Unfortunately it's unlikely you will see a physiotherapist – but for the time being ask your husband to lower your hospital bed as far as possible, which will make it easier for you to get in and out.

YOU'VE DONE IT

Don't worry if you feel spaced out, exhausted, on a high or just thankful it's all over. And you should be feeling pretty pleased with yourself. Your baby (who you secretly know is rather more attractive than anyone else's baby) will be lying in a cot next to your bed. Don't try to do anything but put him to the breast if he cries and close your own eyes if he is asleep.

With any luck, this has been the best day of your life – and the beginning of your new life.

CHAPTER 14

fathers

This chapter is for you. What is said here is distilled from what pregnant women have said to me over time and represents the issues they most frequently say are important. (As some of you will be married and some of you won't be, in an attempt not to antagonise anyone, I randomly refer to the mother of your baby as your partner or your wife.)

Your role as far as your wife and baby are concerned is to provide practical and emotional support – during pregnancy, during labour and during the months with your new baby. This may seem a pretty straightforward statement, but actually long-term (or perhaps seemingly interminable!) support can be hard going, especially as it often seems to go unacknowledged and unappreciated. And because it's the woman who carries your baby, the woman who actually gives birth and (usually) the woman who feeds and cares for your baby, it's difficult for most men not to feel slightly excluded from the whole process. But don't underestimate how much your support is appreciated, even though she probably won't tell you!

PLANNING PATERNITY LEAVE

You may be entitled to up to two weeks' Statutory Paternity Leave with Pay, paid by your employer. You can take this leave any time from your baby's birth up until eight weeks after his due date – but you need to tell your employer at least 15 weeks before you plan to claim paternity leave. Bearing this in mind, it seems sensible to think about all this as early as possible, and to have a discussion with your partner.

The time you will be most needed (and the best time!) is as soon as she and your baby come out of hospital. If you are able to take two full weeks, it might be an idea to split them – allowing a week or so in between for her (or your) mother to help out, and taking the second week when she is on her own again. It is likely that she will be discharged from hospital sooner than you expect. Paternity leave in order for you to provide her with practical and emotional help is no longer a rather idealistic provision but quite a serious business. In London, hospitals now frequently discharge women as early as six hours after having given birth to their first baby. Thirty-odd years ago, women stayed in hospital for 10 days following their first baby, and 48 hours after a second or third baby. (If you don't believe me ask your mothers how long they were in hospital with their first baby.) This means that if you are taking paternity leave in order to look after your wife or partner, you will be caring for someone who is quite definitely not her usual robust self – not ill but in need of some TLC.

You will, of course, know when your baby is due to be born, but it is only an estimated date – babies can be born three weeks before and up to two weeks after their EDD. This leaves you with the slightly tricky problem of not knowing exactly when you will need to take the time off and, if your work allows it, having to keep a month relatively clear so you can be available. Even if you have arranged other help (such as her mother), it is usually best to spend the first day or two as just the three of you together (that's you, your wife and your baby, not you, your wife and her mother). There are two reasons for this. Firstly, it is easier for you as a couple to adjust to having a baby if you have some space for yourselves. Secondly, it means that you, as the father, can get to know your own baby properly and gain confidence in handling him (which you will enjoy!) before other help arrives in the shape of a new grandmother or even a maternity nurse as they tend to want to take over from you.

HOW CAN I HELP MY PARTNER DURING PREGNANCY?

Generally speaking, the support that is really valued during pregnancy is emotional rather than practical. During the process of becoming new parents, you will have some wonderful moments of intense intimacy as well as excitement. But there will also be moments of doubt and apprehension for both of you, and your reassurance and comfort will be much appreciated.

For you, the process of becoming a father is likely to provoke lurking worries of your own, which you probably won't discuss with her:

- Will she and your baby come through OK?
- How will you be able to financially support her *and* a baby?
- Are you going to be any good as a father?
- Will you have to cancel work trips abroad (and risk losing promotion or even your job)?
- Are you ready for all this yet?

Not surprisingly, you will tend to keep these worries to yourself, and you might be wise to do so. Paradoxically, however, this can some-times come across as being uninvolved, and you may find yourself accused of being emotionally removed from the pregnancy, which will seem unfair.

In so many conversations I have had with women during ante-natal classes, they have mentioned that they find it absurdly irritating that their husbands seem uninvolved with their pregnancy and apparently have no idea what it's like being pregnant – all the time. At this point I feel obliged to point out that before becoming preg-nant themselves, they had no idea what it was like and often thought their pregnant girlfriends were making a bit of a fuss about it all. And everyone nods in agreement.

Quite probably, it may seem to you that the woman you fell in love with and is now pregnant seems to have had a total personality change. It is quite normal for women who are pregnant to lose some of their old self-confidence and bounce and become more dependent on you, uncharacteristically indecisive and sometimes tearful – and possibly always tired and sometimes a little irritable. This can mean that however hard you are trying to do the support bit, she may not make it easy for you.

It seems that many men are in danger of being in a no-win situ-ation, but for what it is worth (probably quite a lot), what women tell me they want from you is recognition that:

- pregnancy for some women is not all it's cracked up to be. Many women feel completely different – physically and emotionally – and this is unsettling for them
- they can't 'snap out' of emotional changes and it doesn't mean they don't love you any more

- at the beginning of pregnancy most women feel tired (desperately tired) and possibly nauseated nearly all the time. Getting through a day's work may be bad enough without having to prepare an evening meal
- lethargy is part of pregnancy
- at the end of pregnancy, most women feel increasingly uncomfortable and have to walk slowly. Brisk country walks are out of the question
- a daytime rest, especially at weekends, is not an indulgence but important for your baby
- compliments are more important than ever when your body feels out of control

Essentially, this all comes down to actively maintaining your relationship rather than assuming that it will continue to run along as it has done previously (or even spontaneously take a turn for the better!).

Sharing Domestic Responsibilities

In addition to the huge amount of emotional support your partner needs, you would be really, really appreciated if you could find the time to sit down together and try and re-allocate the division of household tasks whilst she is pregnant. If you don't already do so, it would help if you take on dishwasher packing and unpacking, as by doing this you will save her from getting low backache. If she is going to return to work, the re-allocation of domestic tasks will be permanent, so this is really important to get right now.

One of the biggest issues and grumbles I hear from women is that when they have a baby, they seem to take on the baby as well as everything else – they say they can't face discussing sharing tasks with you and it's easier to do everything themselves! You may think that the fact they don't seem willing to discuss this with you may well be their own fault, and you may be right. However, festering resentment is not exactly an aphrodisiac, so it would seem sensible to try and address this particular issue now.

HOW YOU CAN HELP DURING LABOUR

It's support again – but in order to be able to do this adequately during labour, you need to know the basic anatomy and physiology of what's going on during birth. Therefore it's important that you book into at least one antenatal class, preferably a fathers' evening.

Some men will not want (or be able) to be present at the birth, simply because anything remotely medical makes them feel extremely squeamish or pass out. If you fall into this category, try not to worry that you are already in danger of being a useless father. That is the way you are, and that is the person your partner fell in love with. There is absolutely no evidence that men who are present for the birth of their children make better fathers over the next 30 years. But you will need to take her into hospital and pick her up later at the very least. If you feel that you can't cope with labour itself, it may be worth asking someone else if they would be prepared to come with you so you don't feel pressurised or under stress. One of the important things to realise is that when you take your wife into hospital, you are not 'sucked into the system' and automatically expected to stay the whole time. You can come and go as you (and she) want, and it will be made quite clear when the baby is about to be born, so you can leave then if you want to. You won't have to deliver the baby.

Let's assume that you will take your wife into hospital when she is in labour. With this in mind, it is really important that at some stage during her pregnancy you go together for a hospital tour. This at least means that when you do take her to hospital, you will know where to park the car, whether you need parking money, which door to head for in the middle of the night and which way to turn when you get out of the lift. You will also be able to see what the labour ward looks like. Women in labour are extremely vulnerable and dependent – your wife will certainly not cope well if the car is out of petrol and you are asking her, 'Where exactly is the hospital and how do we get there?'

Another very important issue is for you to work out how to fix the baby's car seat into the car. As women are discharged so early from hospital, your partner might simply not be able to stand for long enough to do this herself.

When Do I Take Her in to Hospital?

First-time mothers generally get to hospital too early so don't try and rush her in at the first contraction. Leave it to her to tell you when she is ready. The only time you need to get her into hospital really quickly is if she is losing fresh blood, or a little less quickly (within about an hour) if her waters have broken.

Otherwise, by rough rules of thumb, she is ready to go to hospital when:

- her contractions are lasting 40 seconds or longer and she has had these contractions for at least two hours
- she feels 'I need my breathing'
- she wants to go in

Some women have several hours (sometimes 12 or more) of early labour (latent stage) which they will spend at home. During this time she will be timing the contractions, starting to practise her breathing during a contraction, working out which positions are most comfortable for her when she has a contraction and probably having a bath or two. Most women are restless in early labour, and it is important that she is able to move around. She can eat and drink what she wants at this stage. You need to be guided by her as to whether she wants you to stay at home with her or would rather you went into work. It goes without saying that if you do go into work, your mobile needs to be on and with you all the time.

Arriving at the Hospital

When you arrive at the hospital, your partner will probably be internally examined by a midwife to see how dilated her cervix is. The midwife might also be able to tell you what position the baby is in, as this helps predict what length of labour you are all in for. With luck she will tell you that the baby is in a favourable position with his head 'well flexed'. You will also both be hoping that your wife is around 3 cm dilated, as many hospitals will send women home if they are less dilated than this. At some stage the baby will be monitored for 40 minutes to check that his heartbeat is doing well.

Going to the Labour Ward

The labour ward is usually a suite of individual rooms and you will be allocated your own midwife. She will stay with you for her shift, which is eight hours. Your most important role is simply to be there; it is your presence that counts. It's a little more than just that of course – it isn't much use if all you do is tackle the crossword or

BlackBerry in silence. Women in labour feel vulnerable and lack self-confidence, and sometimes even lose their ability to ask questions. You are her best friend, and she needs you to lean on for emotional support – and perhaps even to ask the questions!

Practical Things You Can Do

- Help her time the contractions.
- Remind her to start her breathing when a contraction starts (but don't do it with her).
- Remind her to give an audible sigh when the contraction ends.
- Help her to find a position that is comfortable during a contraction – it will be some sort of variation on leaning forwards. Whatever position she can find that makes the contraction easiest to cope with will be the right position.
- Appreciate that most women don't like being touched when they have a contraction, though between contractions she will be her usual self.
- Talk to your midwife! She is on your side, and wants the best for both mother and baby – don't hesitate to ask her about anything you may not understand or are worried about, or for any advice with breathing, positions for labour and so on, even if she seems to spend much of her time writing notes or filling in forms.

If your partner is having trouble relaxing *between* contractions, this is a good indication that she might need pain relief. The best time for an epidural is between 3 cm and 7 cm dilation. If she decides this is what she would like, talk to your midwife who will call for an anaesthetist. Midwives don't give epidurals.

If she is 8 cm dilated or more, she is nearly at the pushing stage and might want to use gas and air (Entonox). Gas and air is usually taken via a mouthpiece – sometimes a mask. It is important that she starts breathing it as deeply as possible at the *beginning* of the contraction, as there is a latent period of around 10–20 seconds before the gas has an effect. Your job is to remind her to stop breathing the gas once she is 10 seconds past the peak of the contraction – this is the most effective way of using it properly (see diagram, page 199).

Most women reach the end of the first stage of labour when their cervix is 10 cm dilated and then simply feel a strong urge to push. Yet some women experience a peculiar change of mood or behaviour at this point known as transition, and you might be alarmed to find her swearing at you and the midwife. It's also not that uncommon for a few women to behave in a seemingly extraordinary way, such as saying 'I'm not having the baby today, I'm going home,' and starting to climb off the bed. This can be coupled with physical symptoms, such as feeling sick, vomiting and sometimes dramatic shivering. One of the problems associated with transition is that your wife may have no insight into the fact that she doesn't have to cope much longer and will therefore need vigorous reassurance. It doesn't last long.

The Second Stage of Labour: Pushing

This is when you are needed at the head end. The midwife will tell your partner when to push, which is during a contraction. If she is in a sitting position, you might want to remind her to:

- drop her chin towards her chest
- think of her diaphragm as the plunger in a cafetière
- 'aim' the baby towards the end of the bed (the midwife may also say 'push into your bottom')

If she is sitting up in bed, it usually helps if, at the beginning of each contraction, you put your hand into her armpit and help her to get back up into a comfortable position as she will tend to slide down the bed when she is pushing.

This stage shouldn't take more than an hour or so, without supervision by an obstetrician – you might want to keep an eye on the clock and ask the midwife for guidance on this. You will know when your baby is about to be born as the staff will put on gloves and a mask and open a sterile pack.

When the baby's head is born, the midwife will ask the mother to 'pant'. Your wife may not register this, so check that she has heard the midwife's instructions. When your baby is born, the midwife might ask whether you would like to cut the baby's cord. This is entirely up to you – there will be no long-term effect on your relationship with your baby if you do or don't cut his cord.

If your baby needs an 'assisted delivery' (forceps or ventouse) and if your wife needs stitches afterwards, stay at the head end. She will be put in the 'lithotomy' position (legs in stirrups).

A Caesarean Delivery – Emergency or Elective

It might be that labour doesn't progress as straightforwardly as it should and the medical staff decide that your baby needs to be delivered by Caesarean section. Or your partner may have been booked in for an elective Caesarean section. Whatever the reason, if you can face sitting with her while your baby is delivered, it will be really reassuring for her. If you were going to have a Caesarean, you too would appreciate your best friend being there with you. Nearly all Caesarean sections are given under local anaesthetic (epidural), but in the unlikely event that she needs a general anaesthetic, you will not be present.

Most Caesarean deliveries are carried out in the hospital theatre, which may be on a different floor to the delivery room. A theatre is a chain of three rooms – an ante-room where the anaesthetist administers or tops up an epidural; the theatre where the operation takes place; and the recovery room where the patient is looked after before going down to the ward.

When your wife goes into the theatre, there will be an anaesthetist sitting on one side and you will sit on the other side, so you (and the anaesthetist) can chat to her. There will be a screen just below her chest so you won't see anything! The operating staff will be 'gowned up', meaning they will be in theatre gear in order to keep things as sterile as possible, and wearing gowns, sterile boots (not because they will be wading through anything), hats, gloves and masks. You will also be given a gown and a hat to wear for the same reason. It will take a very short time (about 10–15 minutes) to deliver your baby, who will be passed over the screen to your wife, and she will probably soon pass him over to you to hold. It takes perhaps a surprisingly long time to sew her up again, but at this stage you will probably be rather taken by your baby – and your wife will want (and need) to gaze at him while she is being tidied up. When the placenta has been delivered and she has been stitched up again, you will be moved to the recovery room.

Don't be alarmed when you see that she seems to be attached to quite a few tubes:

- an epidural catheter over her shoulder
- probably a drip in the back of her hand
- a catheter draining wee from her bladder into a bottle fixed to the side of the bed
- probably a drain to take fluid from the horizontal incision in her lower abdomen, also draining into another bottle

All these tubes will be removed over the next day or so.

All three of you will stay in the recovery room for an hour or so while the staff check that her blood pressure is OK. When the epidural wears off, they will give her alternative pain relief. As soon as the staff are happy that she is stable, you will be transferred to the postnatal ward.

Directly after the Birth

Seeing your own baby being born is a powerful and wonderful experience. New babies are good news. You may be surprised to find that you are rather more moved than your partner – it is not unusual to find the father in emotional tears but the mother simply asking for a cup of tea. If this is the case, it doesn't mean she hasn't 'bonded'. Hospitals are well aware that you as a couple need to be alone quietly with your baby for an hour or so, and they try and cater for this. At this stage you need to remember:

- Your wife may be anxious about holding the baby and generally getting things right (even if she works with babies herself).
- She will probably be exhausted, and if she has a drip in the back of her hand will find holding the baby awkward – if she has had a Caesarean it may be really difficult.

- Babies have a strong suckling reflex in the first hour after birth, so she will probably be encouraged to put the baby to the breast, which will help 'kick-start' her production of milk.

GETTING IT RIGHT AFTERWARDS

This is much more practical support. You don't necessarily need to take the whole day off if your wife is staying in hospital for a couple of nights, but you do need to arrange a short working day, as you will want to see her in the evenings. While she is in hospital, your role is to:

- Keep the house extremely clean – women who have just had babies are often a bit funny about cleanliness.
- Do any washing for her.
- Shop for food – even if she is having her baby at a private hospital, she will need extra provisions.
- Make an awful lot of phone calls, texts and emails to let people know the news (her mother is conventionally the first to hear).
- Ensure unexpected visitors don't turn up at the hospital – the only people she has to see are you and perhaps both sets of what are now grandparents.

When you collect your new family from the hospital, take the baby's car seat up to the ward. You will already have worked out how to fix the baby's car seat into the car (see above), but you will now need to work out how to fix the baby into the car seat. The shoulder straps go *over* the shoulders, and it's a little tricky getting the crutch strap between the legs of a swaddled baby. All this is much easier to work out calmly in your own time while your wife is getting dressed, rather than trying to do it in the car park in the rain. When you leave the hospital together, you will need to remember that women who have had a baby can only walk slowly, and women who have had a baby by Caesarean section can only walk very slowly indeed.

Take mother and baby home to a spotlessly clean, tidy and empty house. There are three things that you will be responsible for when she gets home:

- making sure she gets some sleep during the day
- monitoring visitors (again)
- buying and preparing meals

It is very important that your wife has what used to be called a 'lying-in period'. This means she should be in night-gear and in or near her bed for the first 10 days after the birth. This is necessary in order that she recovers from the physical impact of the birth, gets lactation established and falls into step with your baby. Many women have a 'high' during the first few days following childbirth so getting her to change into a nightdress and stay in bed could present a bit of a problem for you. It might be worth bearing in mind that the more rest she gets in the early weeks, the quicker her long-term recovery will be, which will obviously be in your interest as well as hers. Perhaps surprisingly, most women are at their most tired when their baby is around 10 weeks old.

Visitors are a major problem. On a survey my practice did a few years back, we asked women to write down what their husbands did that was most and least helpful following childbirth. Top of the lists by far of the most helpful things was monitoring family and visitors. You need to give them an 'appointment' which is not at a time when your wife usually has a sleep, and make sure they don't stay too long; half an hour is about right. If they bring their own children (who always seem to have a cold) make sure they don't breathe all over your baby! The other advantage of your wife being in a nightdress is that it will remind visitors that she has just had a baby and is not yet up to entertaining.

Organising the meals should be reasonably straightforward, except you will find you seem to be food shopping more than usual. You will need to organise breakfast, lunch, tea (cakes or biscuits) and supper. This is probably much more than she was used to eating in the office, but it is usual for women who have had babies to feel continuously thirsty and hungry and to crave sugar, especially if they are breastfeeding. On this subject, it's probably best if you avoid adding garlic to her food for the first few weeks as it can sometimes make babies uncomfortable. The other adjustment is the time of your evening meal. She will really appreciate it (and you!) if you can aim to get supper ready early – probably around 7pm. This is much better for her than an elaborate gourmet meal at 9pm with the best claret and the candelabra.

A woman who has just had a baby is intensely vulnerable, lacking in self-confidence and often overwhelmed by the sheer responsibility of looking after something so helpless and precious. This is at a time when she is not exactly feeling fighting fit herself. Not only has she to recover from the process of labour, but if her labour stretched over a couple of nights, she (and you) may be seriously sleep-deprived already. Added to this, it is likely that she will have sore stitches, and when her breasts produce milk on the third or fourth day, painful breasts. She needs loads of positive feedback and encouragement from you – especially if any initial attempts at breastfeeding don't seem to be going well. Stay positive and avoid making any helpful suggestions that can easily be perceived as critical. If you absolutely have to, start your comment with something like, 'Wouldn't it be a good idea...' rather than, 'Why don't you...' or 'What you should do...' Tolerate the uncertainty of your new life with patience. One of the over-riding challenges of the first week with a new baby is working out why he cries and what to do about it.

Perhaps one other thing to remember: she needs you more than she has ever needed you before, even if it seems to you that she only cares about your baby. The first few weeks with your first baby will be amazing and wonderful, and both of you will discover reserves of energy and things about yourself and each other that you never knew you had. These weeks are pivotal with regard to your future life together. And you, of course, will be anxious to get things right.

CONCLUSION

you as a new mother

I DON'T LIKE BABIES VERY MUCH – WHAT IF I DON'T LIKE MINE?

This is quite a common secret worry – 'Oh my God, I'm going to be the only woman in the world who doesn't fall in love with her own baby and it's going to be so embarrassing.' As it happens, you will fall in love with him, though quite a few women don't do so immediately, and sometimes not for many weeks.

One of the most helpful things about having second- or third-time mothers in antenatal classes is that I can ask them what their reaction was when they first saw their baby, and how long it took before they fell in love with him. This is riveting information to the first-time mothers – I can see some of them almost hold their breath with fascination. I guess this means that quite a few have been worried about this. The responses from different mothers are always interesting. Firstly, the good news is that I haven't had anyone who said they *never* fell in love with their baby. In fact, when they are talking about the child they now have, they all say they love them so much they would willingly die for them. There is a separate issue here – many mothers who are pregnant with their third child say, 'Actually, I love my other two so desperately, now I'm expecting a third baby I'm a bit worried if I've got enough love to go round.' (You will have!)

From what I have heard, about 60 per cent of women say that they fell in love with their baby at first sight, which may be rather less than some would otherwise assume. They often say, 'I wasn't expecting it, but I was totally besotted as soon as he was put into my arms.' Some mothers (about 35 per cent) say it happens a few days later, and it can be literally just the same as falling in love with a guy – extraordinarily powerful, completely overwhelming and of course wonderful! The sort of things they say are: 'They gave him to me and I looked at him and thought, oh…he looks just like my father-in-law.' Or, 'Well, I felt absolutely knackered. I didn't *not* like him but I felt totally spaced out and overwhelmed with the responsibility of keeping him alive. I just didn't really feel very much else. It was only when I came home that it hit me how totally wonderful he was.' But for about 5 per cent of women, the falling in love doesn't happen for several weeks or sometimes as long as a few months later, even if they thought they had a close bond with their baby during pregnancy, and felt sure there would be an instant love between them.

There may be understandable reasons for not falling in love with your baby until later, such as being exhausted, in pain, disappointed that your birth wasn't what you expected, or frightened that your baby wasn't going to be OK. But sometimes there are no reasons – that's just the way it is. However, new babies are good news, and you certainly won't find yours disgusting or not want to touch him – apart from anything else, your own baby smells quite delicious! Yes really! And babies are programmed to make their mothers fall in love with them at some stage – they have to do this because they are so helpless and dependent and incapable of surviving on their own.

Bonding

Whoever delivers your baby will be anxious to get things right for you. Some midwives think that it's important for your baby to be placed onto your tummy (before the cord is cut) in order for you to get skin-to-skin contact as soon as possible. Although some (not all) studies have shown that a new mother who has skin-to-skin contact with her baby is a little more likely to succeed with breastfeeding, this is by no means crucial. It also used to be said (wrongly) that skin-to-skin contact at the time of delivery was essential for mother and baby to 'bond' but this is now known not to be true. You don't have to have your baby naked on your tummy, or anywhere else if you don't want to. If you want your baby wrapped up before you hold him, that's also perfectly normal! You don't have to 'bond' with your baby immediately in order for your relationship over the next 30 years to be fulfilling, in spite of what you may be told. Try not to worry – if you don't fall in love with your baby at first, relax and let things take their time. He won't know, and you won't have FAILURE TO BOND stamped over your hospital notes.

At some stage, you will fall in love with him – and he will fall in love with you.

INDEX

A Perfect Start
Christine and Peter Hill

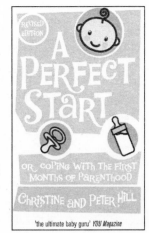

The perfect guide to helping new parents survive the early months of caring for a newborn baby.

For many parents the first few months after a baby's birth can be a time of shock and adjustment as well as personal joy. In this friendly, accessible guide, Christine and Peter Hill provide a vast amount of practical and down-to-earth guidance on:

- How to cope with persistent crying
- Dealing with feelings of depression and isolation
- Looking after yourself as well as your baby
- How to maintain fulfilling relationships with parents and friends
- When and when not to return to work

9780091917425 £8.99

What to Expect When You're Breast-feeding... and What If You Can't?
Clare Byam-Cook

An invaluable guide with clear and sensible advice for new mothers.

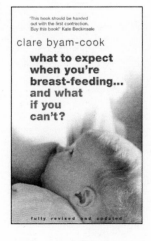

This comprehensive guide has been fully revised and updated to contain all the latest information on breast-feeding your baby successfully, including how to prepare, what to expect in the early stages and how to overcome common problems. And rather than making you feel guilty if you prefer, or have to, bottle feed, Clare Byam-Cook is wholly supportive and sympathetic, providing you with all the practical advice and information you need.

9780091906962 £8.99

FREE POSTAGE AND PACKING
Overseas customers allow £2.00 per paperback.

ORDER:

By phone: 01624 677237

By post: Random House Books
c/o Bookpost
PO Box 29
Douglas
Isle of Man IM99 1BQ

By fax: 01624 670923

By email: bookshop@enterprise.net

Cheques (payable to Bookpost) and credit cards accepted.

Prices and availability subject to change without notice.
Allow 28 days for delivery.
When placing your order, please mention if you do not
wish to receive any additional information.

www.rbooks.co.uk